You Tell Them:
"It's In Their Head"

YOU TELL THEM: "IT'S IN THEIR HEAD"

Personal Health Stories

Narrated and Commented On By
James Scala, Ph.D.

Frontrunner Books

FRONTRUNNER BOOKS
Published and exclusively distributed by:
Frontrunner Books
1820 Homestead Trail,
Long Lake, Minnesota 55356-9352, U.S.A.

NOTE TO THE READER

The ideas, procedures, and suggestions contained in this book are not intended as a substitute for consulting with your physician. All matters regarding your health require medical supervision.

FOR ADDITIONAL SINGLE OR QUANTITY ORDERS, CALL/WRITE:
FRONTRUNNERS BOOKS, 1820 HOMESTEAD TRAIL, LONG LAKE, MINNESOTA 55356-9352.
TOLL FREE: (800) 237-5199
FAX: (612) 475-3715

To: Forrest C. Shaklee, Sr.
A plain spoken man whose gift of inspiration
helped many people realize their dreams.

——J.S.

Acknowledgments

A few dedicated people helped me complete this book, with both their insight and hard work. Special thanks go to:

Nancy Scala, my wife and partner, for her thoughts, typing, and editing.

Kimberly Scala, my daughter, for her typing, comments, and willingness to assist.

Mary Loomis, a dear friend, for reading the manuscript, her suggestions, and support.

And to all those people whose wonderful health stories made this book possible.

Contents

This is not a book of medical cures

For fourteen years, I have collected these vignettes on my travels . They do not represent clinical research, medical practice, or cures. In no way should anyone use them as a guide to substitue for medical care, counsel, or advice. The interpretations are mine and do not necessarily represent scientific consensus. No endorsement was sought by any corporation, none is expected, and none is implied.

——J.S.

Introduction

For the last 14 years, I've had the good fortune to meet some very determined people with serious physical ailments. This book tells how they overcame many obstacles, and either solved or managed their health problems with nutrition when other approaches had failed to give them the quality of life they wanted. Some of these people were confronted with the prospects of life as a cripple, being dependent on heavy medication, or both.

Doctor Shaklee once told me I'd hear about these unusual experiences and to be prepared to listen politely. For several years, that's exactly how I reacted, but slowly I began to realize that these stories were too consistent to be imagined or made up. Too many people had comparable experiences, tried the same things, and had similar results. Either the stories were real or I was witness to some strange, mass hysteria. I resolved to listen more carefully.

It became obvious that there is a similarity about the people with these illnesses. I don't mean they all look or dress alike, or go to the same church, but I detected an inner sameness. They had an individual glow that was evident, but hard to describe. Indeed, some of these people could barely get around because they were so crippled or in constant pain, but each one had a smile that you couldn't wipe away. They also had the kind of silent confidence you see in great leaders; you might not accept their belief or persuasion, but you can sense their integrity.

Physically, these people were as different as any group could be: some were short, some tall, some overweight, and others looked like a good wind could blow them away. Some had extensive education and others exaggerated when they claimed an eighth-grade education. I met medical doctors from the best universities and people educated in the humanities. Some were successful performers and others had never left the farm. When they all got together, there were no barriers, because they shared a common ground of mutual respect. They had all achieved a level of health that had previously eluded them.

Every man and woman among them was devoted to Doctor Shaklee and his products. Some of them sold the products, built large businesses, and had excellent incomes. Others used the products and shared them with a few close friends at their cost, so they made very little money, if any, after expenses. And still others simply bought the products for their own personal use. I ruled out economic interest in the products, because most of these people didn't sell enough products to cover their expenses. I also noticed that they had a way of referring to Doctor Shaklee simply as "Doctor," in a sort of reverent tone, so you knew exactly who they were talking about. Few leaders ever have that kind of loyal following.

I asked myself why I kept listening? I discussed these stories with professional friends and always heard the same comments expressed in several ways. "It's all in their head," was the most common comment. One day I heard that comment once too often and said, "You better tell them that, because some of them don't realize they can't walk, or aren't on drugs, or don't stutter, or didn't die!" Now that I can look back on the experience, I realize that my thinking had expanded. Few people are privileged to grow in that way.

MY MIND WAS PREPARED

Over the years I had always paid close attention to old wives' tales or, more correctly, folklore about health. In 1955 through 1968, I read a series of papers which, taken together, explained the incredible accuracy and health value of the old saying "every child needs the January sun." It was hard to believe this saying was well established by the 13th century. It was attributed to women who simply passed health information on from one generation to the other through these sayings. This wisdom could have prevented a lot of suffering and death in the 18th, 19th and 20th centuries if people had followed it then. It took us until 1921 to fortify milk with vitamin D and end suffering from rickets. Women in the 13th century simply used sunlight to accomplish the same thing.

During the late 1960s, I followed the teachings of Dennis Burkitt and realized that his research papers on fiber were 20th-century proof of observations first recognized by Hippocrates, that later emerged in England as the old wives' tale, "an apple a day keeps the doctor away." Consequently, I wrote a paper entitled "Fiber: The Forgotten Nutrient," which was published for my writing quality and not its scientific content. At the time, the journal referees said fiber simply wasn't an important topic. If health policymakers had paid more attention to the basis of that old wives' tale, our health-care costs would be much lower today.

Without realizing it, I had fallen into a trap which Louis Pasteur would have predicted when he said, "Chance favors the mind that's prepared." My interest in folklore and the respect I developed for folk wisdom had prepared my mind to accept what I heard. It became apparent that I was hearing folklore in the making when I heard all these stories. It brought to mind a comment Doctor Shaklee had made one day in the lab while our conversation was being filmed: "Making a discovery is easy. It's knowing a discovery has been made that's difficult." How right he was.

EXPERIENCES HAVE AN IMPORTANT PLACE

Old wives' tales are solid because they have stood the test of time. People make observations and pass them from one generation to the next. If they're valid, they get passed again and again and finally emerge as folk remedies. This is how people discovered the effects of garlic, aspirin, colchicine, a drug for gout, Epsom salts, feverfew, milk of magnesia, and many other remedies and drugs that are here today. More importantly, many of them, such as the omega-3 oils and even beta carotene, have been rediscovered, thanks to the folklore that had grown up around them.

I've used representative stories that are typical of many that I've heard. This book is not a scientific analysis. Within these stories, I believe there's a lot of grist for future research. This is consistent with the health sciences, where much research began as anecdotal stories that gave an inquisitive scientist an idea.

We've all experienced these interesting incidents in the last two decades with the book *Life After Life* by Raymond A. Moody, M.D. Doctor Moody heard about experiences by patients who had been declared dead, but were brought back. All the stories had a sameness to them and it didn't matter what the background of the person was from an educational, religious, or ethnic standpoint. Besides, the people were convinced and had an inner glow about their experience. You couldn't tell them it was in their head.

Dr. Moody decided there was something to these stories and he had to tell people about them. When I read his book, I admit I was skeptical, but over the years other scientists began to take notice and did some additional studies. In 1990, the phenomenon was so well established that Melvin Morse, M.D. published his book *Closer To The Light*, which is as valid a scientific study as you'll ever find and focuses only on the near-death experiences of children. He chose children because they were too innocent to lie. Morse's studies proved Moody was correct. So, in spite of the early skeptics, we are faced with an entirely new aspect of our conscious mind. What is most interesting about these experiences is that as far back as we can accurately document human occurrences (that's over 3,000 years), people have said the same thing! All Raymond Moody did was tell the world, so someone could give it the attention it deserves.

ARTHRITIS

"You only think you're getting better. Diet can't help arthritis! Sure, you feel better when you follow the diet and take vitamins, but it isn't that they are doing anything for you, it's because you're doing something for yourself. That's why we call it a placebo effect. For now, I want you to continue with this program, but we'll start the gold injections and get this under control."

Mildred's doctor spoke with such certainty that she questioned her own feelings. The swelling in her hands and ankles was bad, the pain was intense, the medication made her feel sick to her stomach, and she had dizzy spells and a rash. Her doctor said her arthritis was in the early stages and his plan was to try and stop its progress. She remembered how her mother suffered with arthritis and those awful gold shots she had to get for so many years. As these thoughts drifted through her mind, she recalled how she had started the diet and supplements.

She decided to follow a diet her neighbor told her about, along with the medicine she was taking. The diet was hard to follow because she had to eat fish and cutout meat and dairy products. Her husband had to have his beef, so it meant cooking two meals every night. Although the diet plan was hard for her to follow, after about three weeks or a month, she seemed to feel better and the swelling wasn't as bad. In fact, she could do housework again and even went to some of the coffee klatches her friends had. At the same time, she took the terrible fish-oil capsules with their "fishy" aftertaste and those big green vitamin-pills her friend sold her.

Then her daughter Connie and her husband had marital problems. She knew it was coming, but had hoped that somehow they would work it out. Connie and the children came home to live, which upset Mildred's diet plan. With the added responsibility of caring for her three grandchildren so Connie could go back to her old job, Mildred often forgot to take her supplements. Shortly after, she woke up one morning with her hands and ankles all red and puffy and hurting like the dickens. The pain and swelling kept getting worse throughout the day. Her husband insisted she go to the doctor and told her, as he had often done before, that the diet and all the vitamins were nonsense. After much arguing, Connie agreed that she should see the doctor. After all, he was an expert and, she had to admit, her neighbor was just selling the supplements. So, here she was, right back at square one! Right where she had been 30 years ago.

Conversations similar to this take place a million times a year in thousands of doctor's offices all over the country. Although the woman in this vignette swears she felt better and looked better than she had in a long time, she got argued down. Mildred would have to be a strong person, with lots of positive supporters around her, to stay with a diet and the supplements. This is because it takes nutrition time to work; in this case, six months. Unfortunately, diet and supplement plans are easy to stop when you're the only one in the family on them. Nutrition is teamwork among nutrients, and among people.

Don't get the idea that Mildred's doctor had anything but the best intentions for her, because he did. He had simply been programmed by a system that, since about 1930, says diet can't help arthritis. In fact, the Arthritis Foundation has emphasized this position to such a degree, that to think otherwise until May 1990, was to be looked upon as a heretic. Consequently, the doctor follows the course that is prescribed by the "experts." This course is to use even stronger medication to reduce the symptoms, so the arthritis patient can be as free of pain as possible. There's no such thing as a cure for this disease.

If Mildred's doctor had read a paper by Dr. E. D. Harris in the May 3, 1990 issue of the most widely read of all medical journals, *The New England Journal of Medicine*, he might have acted more openly. Dr. Harris' paper explains that diet is appropriate therapy for stages two and three of rheumatoid arthritis – that's when there's swelling in the joints, but no serious loss of cartilage (Mildred's stage). At stage four, when cartilage loss is noticeable, it's no longer appropriate. He goes on to explain how a diet of fish, no meat etc., and the use of fish-oil supplements can be an excellent approach at these stages. Harris' paper goes on to explain the mechanisms by which the diet and supplements work. Diet and supplements can be used effectively to treat arthritis!

How many people were told for years that diet and supplements are a waste of time and money? How many of these people that followed the standard course, would love to go back in time and start over? How many doctors, that read Harris' paper, thought back to all their patients that asked if diet could help them, and remember saying "it's nonsense"? Worse yet, how many people called the Arthritis Foundation and asked for information, only to receive a brochure saying that a balanced diet was the only way to go, because diet couldn't help? A footnote to this story concerns the "gold" shots that are still used with regularity for arthritis. Research has proven that they are ineffective after three years, even though many people have been getting them regularly for ten years. But more research has proven that they are no better than some common anti-inflammatory medications that have, by comparison, very minor side-effects.

IT'S NOT IN YOUR HEAD

Mildred is an example of what I want to accomplish in this book. I know that her relief from the diet and supplements was real and not in her head. Now I have the authority of *The New England Journal of Medicine* as my support. She had none. She took the least resistant, if not the most devastating course, and stuck with the whole gamut of drugs as her only treatment. Today Mildred is a cripple; her hands are so bad you don't like to look at them; she needs a cane to walk; and pain is her constant companion. Things like a quick trip to the store would be a real luxury for her. I can't say that she could have avoided this end result, but she could have probably delayed it and saved herself from the side effects of many drugs.

THE PEOPLE IN THIS BOOK

This is a book about special people who were told that diet and supplements are nonsense, but they prevailed. When experts or friends said it was in their head, they said, "Okay, but until my head says differently, I'm sticking with my nutritional plan." They stuck with it, so now some can walk, even though they were told they wouldn't; some can do things they were told would be impossible because of a bad heart; others are alive because they licked a deadly disease.

Other people in this book had an illness that was seemingly impossible for doctors to deal with, and they exhausted all options to no avail. Then, usually out of desperation, they turned to nutrition and succeeded. You'll meet a stutterer who doesn't stutter; arthritics who can walk; people with multiple sclerosis and epilepsy who got out of their wheelchairs. All of these individuals have two things in common: they stuck with nutrition, and the word "quit" isn't in their vocabulary.

You Tell Them: "It's In Their Head"

CHAPTER

1 AIDS

DAVE'S STORY

" 'You're HIV positive!' The words cut like a knife. At first, I didn't want to believe it. I couldn't have AIDS. It was a mistake; take another test," was Dave's reaction, as he told me about his situation. "Then, reality set in. You have to get on with your life. After all, some HIV-positive people never get symptoms of AIDS for years."

Dave is in excellent condition. He's a physical conditioner by avocation and a graphic artist by profession. He had noticed a modest weight loss, some sore throats and colds. He wondered: Could this be the beginning?

Dave's doctor did an analysis of his immune system. Specifically, he had a "T" cell count done. His "T" cells came back at a level of 480. That number is below the 500 cut off at which an HIV-positive person would be put on the drug AZT. (A normal "T" cell count is 1,000 for someone whose immune system is fine.) However, they decided to wait and see if his nutrition program would improve the situation.

Dave had started a nutrition plan that included Vita-Lea, B-Complex, vitamin C, EPA, vitamin E, Formula I, calcium-magnesium, Performance, and Physique. Within a month, he had gained back his lost weight. He had a second blood test taken and his "T" cell level was 490. The trend was pointing in the right direction. His doctor said it was better to put off AZT as long as possible. So, they agreed that Dave should keep the nutrition program going and have another blood test taken in a month. He did. The next "T" cell level was 540! Comfortably above the 500 cut off for AZT, so the doctor simply said: "Let's leave well enough alone." Dave is still not on AZT.

"If I miss something in my nutrition program, I start dragging," Dave said with alacrity. "It's as if I need a powerful nutrition program just to keep up with my needs. At first I thought it was my aggressive fitness program, but then I realized something else was going on. Now I realize that my tiredness was from the AIDS." I told Dave that his conclusion is probably correct. Although there's no direct proof in his case, research supports his intuition.

Five people test HIV positive every two hours in the United States. It's one of the worst diseases we have ever had to face in this country, if not the world. People who test positive must continue with their lives under the cloud of impending health deterioration, and must face an early death. It's a dreadful disease.

One of the first signs of AIDS that goes unnoticed is a decline in the health of cells that line the small intestines. This change causes a decline in the absorption of nutrients. Consistent with a decline in absorptive capacity, recent research indicates that HIV-positive people are deficient in several nutrients: zinc, several B-vitamins, and choline, which is obtained from lecithin. These nutrition-related findings explain why, in Africa where AIDS originated, folklore refers to AIDS as "the slimming disease." The earliest symptom a person could observe was weight loss, a general slimming. This slimming was accompanied by no apparent symptoms, so the simple folk name is very descriptive. Much later, the victim would develop horrible symptoms as other AIDS-related diseases started to increase.

A decline in absorptive capacity, malabsorption, leaves only one option: get more nutrients. The only practical way to get more nutrients is by supplementing with vitamins, minerals, and protein, which give the body its building blocks to keep the immune system up and tissue repair going. It's also essential to eat a balanced diet with lots of carbohydrates; a little fat in the diet is probably all right for folks with AIDS.

Dave's approach to fighting AIDS, and the success he experienced, is consistent with what science has uncovered about AIDS. I urged him to keep his program going and, if anything, to increase his supplement use. Besides following a good nutrition plan, Dave also maintains his fitness program and his graphic-arts work. I look forward to hearing about his progress for many years to come.

CHAPTER

2 Arthritis

JEANETTE'S STORY

"I couldn't get out of bed. I thought my knees were on fire.
Nothing like the ache I would get sometimes." Jeanette
talks about it like it was yesterday and not 22 years ago.
"I remember the doctor saying I had rheumatoid arthritis.
The first thought that went through my mind was that
rheumatoid arthritis is something old people get. I was
only 22."

Jeanette started with large quantities of aspirin which
seemed to help, but her knees and hands continued swelling off and on, so the doctor prescribed stronger medication. The pain would subside for awhile, but if the
weather changed or got cold, it would come back. Then,
when Jeanette got pregnant, things began to change.

"While I was pregnant, the swelling and pain disappeared. I wished I could always be pregnant, but without
having lots of babies. I love children, but the arthritis
seemed to get worse after I stopped nursing. It was almost
like the arthritis was making up for lost time," she said,

while wringing her hands. Her knuckles were large and
knobby, a characteristic of rheumatoid arthritis. I could
see that discussing her problem made her uncomfortable.

WHAT IS ARTHRITIS?

Rheumatoid arthritis is an inflammatory autoimmune
disease that attacks the joints, usually the knees, hips, and
hands. However, some types of arthritis attack the back
and neck. This disease has a definite hereditary history
and usually appears in the female side of a family. Consequently, about three out of four people with rheumatoid
arthritis are women.

In spite of the hereditary factor, most experts suspect
a viral origin. It seems that in some people a viral infection in early life, such as a case of flu or mononucleosis,
is required. It's theorized that the virus remains dormant
in the membrane that surrounds the joints and holds in the
fluid that lubricates them. This membrane is named the
synovial membrane and the fluid is the synovial fluid.

Some form of severe stress, physical or emotional,
starts the dormant virus growing. Two things happen under stress: body temperature often drops, and the immune
system declines. Both changes favor the growth of dormant viruses. That's why people often catch cold or flu
when they are run down, tired, or there's a family tragedy. When the virus in the joint starts growing, the body
starts a defense strategy in motion. First, it causes the
joint to become inflamed and the immune system sends in
cells to attack the virus. Unfortunately, it's thought that
these cells attack cells in the synovial membrane. To
counter this attack, the synovial membrane grows more

rapidly than normal. Excessive membrane growth causes the membrane to become highly convoluted. These convolutions increase the tissue in and around the joint, causing it to become distorted. Each flare-up makes the membrane grow a little more and the joint becomes a little worse, until it's permanently swollen, distorted, and not very functional. The only approach to restoring functionality is surgery, which often includes a joint replacement.

I suggest you purchase my book entitled *The Arthritis Relief Diet* in which I discuss some of the 375 arthritis cases that I studied. The book explains the types of physical and emotional stress that trigger flare-ups and the methods employed to stop them.

Arthritis in women is often dormant during pregnancy. Jeanette is a typical example. This dormancy probably results from the normal changes that occur during pregnancy that have an effect on the activity of the immune system. The remission usually lasts as long as the mother nurses her infant. Sometimes a woman will have mild arthritis and, following pregnancy, the disease will start up again with a vengeance. Sometimes the baby can go home, but the mother can't.

Like all inflammatory diseases, arthritis can go into remission, even in advanced stages, and then flare up again. A flare-up is usually traceable to some form of stress, either physical or mental. Examples of physical stress include a serious chill, a significant change in the weather, excessive fatigue, or a serious fall, to name a few. Emotional stress includes divorce, a serious argument, illness, the death of a loved one, problems with the children, and so on. If you can think of something that will disrupt a person's life, it can probably elicit an arthritis flare-up.

In recent years, experts have recognized that certain foods can cause flare-ups. Folklore has claimed this fact for generations, but it was largely ignored. In my book, I cite many examples of these antagonistic foods, that range from some plant foods to many animal foods, such as beef and dairy products. There are no firm rules on which foods are causative. Consequently, a thorough on-going food-diary is the only way to identify these food sensitivities if you have arthritis. I emphasize that these reactions to food are sensitivities and not allergies. If you're allergic to a certain food, eating just a little bit of it will cause a response. With a sensitivity, the response is much slower and can sometimes take several days before it affects you.

Arthritis can strike at any age, even juveniles under the age of two. A minor consolation is that young children usually seem to outgrow the disease. When it strikes after puberty, it's often permanent.

There are two general types of arthritis: osteo and rheumatoid. Osteoarthritis affects the bones only and seems to be part of any animal with a skeleton. We'll all get osteoarthritis if we live long enough. In contrast, rheumatoid arthritis affects only the soft tissue and is the arthritis we are discussing here. Rheumatoid arthritis has as many as a hundred variations.

RETURN TO JEANETTE

"My arthritis seemed to get progressively worse. Our family doctor sent me to a rheumatologist who used steroids during a flare-up. The first few days after the steroid injections I felt terrible and couldn't sleep, but once the side effects wore off, I felt good again. I used prescription analgesics daily to keep the pain and swelling down. During one particularly long flare-up, my rheumatologist suggested I try gold shots."

Gold shots are injections of a salt from the metal gold. They are usually given monthly and are moderately painful because a large needle is necessary. The side affects of gold shots can be devastating. These side effects range from a mild rash, which usually disappears in a few weeks, to death, and a number of problems in between. Only 50 percent of the people who start gold shots can continue. During the first three months of gold shots, the patient is monitored weekly. This weekly monitoring is necessary to detect a reaction.

DID THEY WORK?

"At first I felt that the shots were worse than the arthritis, but the side effects subsided and I felt better. My arthritis didn't seem to flare up, but it kept progressing. At least I didn't take any more drugs," she said. "Then my life changed."

"A friend, Connie, had attended a Shaklee nutrition seminar where a woman spoke on how supplements helped her arthritis. This friend had gotten her name and suggested I speak with her. She offered to take me to see this lady," she said, and quickly continued to explain why.

"By this time, I couldn't get around very well. My knees were always swollen and my hands were getting knobby. My friends could tell that I hurt a lot and they wanted to do something. I was very tired and took naps regularly. If it weren't for our two children, I know my husband would have left. I felt bad for him because he had a good job and I know I was holding him back. Our sex life was over partly because of my pain and partly because of my appearance. I had discussed these problems with Connie and she was trying to help. So, I agreed to go, as much for her as for me."

Jeanette explained why she didn't put much hope in Connie's effort. "I had read all the information on arthritis. It emphatically said that diet and nutrition had no effect on the disease. All the literature advised was to eat a well-balanced diet."

Up to this point, Jeanette maintained a wholesome diet. Neither she nor her family used supplements regularly. Like many people, she purchased supplements in the drugstore from time to time and would use them off and on. As often as not, she and her husband would use the supplement for awhile, and then they would collect dust somewhere in the kitchen or medicine cabinet. Visiting the home of an enthusiastic Shaklee user was an experience for Jeanette.

"We were greeted at Helen's door with a spirited smile. I could tell immediately from her hands that her arthritis had progressed beyond mine, but it didn't seem to slow her down. She had a gleam in her eye and seemed to be full of energy. We laughed a lot that morning. Her enthusiasm was infectious. I felt good just being with her. Connie and I sat down and she told me her story."

Helen explained how her arthritis had progressed similar to Jeanette's. It started shortly after her messy divorce was final and continued with a vengeance. She said the divorce was her husband's doing, but she thought she was being punished when she got arthritis. She had gone the same drug route as Jeanette had gone, except she wouldn't take the gold shots when her doctor proposed them. She decided to try an alternate approach. She tried several things, but the nutrition was the only one that worked. Though, she added, that meditation seemed to help a great deal.

Jeanette was shocked at the suggestion of taking 35 alfalfa tablets. Instant Protein in juice was all right, and she could handle taking more supplements than she knew existed, but alfalfa was animal food and 35 tablets of anything seemed excessive. In her own words, she decided to try, for a simple reason. "I decided that if I could have half of Helen's energy and outlook, I'd be willing to take twice as much alfalfa." She quickly added, "I didn't care if my hair turned green from the alfalfa, and I had to stick with the gold shots."

Jeanette will be the first to explain that it wasn't easy to take all the supplements. She gagged on the alfalfa, tasted fish from the EPA, and felt bloated to the point of bursting from the protein. Let her tell you what happened.

"One morning, after about ten days of this, I realized it was 10:00 o'clock. I had been up since 7:00 A.M. and didn't even give a thought to a nap. In fact, I planned to go shopping and hadn't even realized how good I felt. I wanted to tell everyone, but decided to tell my doctor."

Jeanette's doctor was skeptical about nutrition, but he couldn't ignore her enthusiasm and the fact that she looked better than he could ever remember. Consequently, they agreed to work together to overcome her problem. In a period of six months, she got herself off the gold shots and settled on a prescription, non-steroid, anti-inflammatory drug. She used this drug whenever she felt pain or inflammation. "After all," she said, "I can avoid lots of things, but not the weather or my kids."

Now, years later, she still uses the supplements regularly. In her own words, "I haven't felt this good since my first child. Our personal life is active again. With our children close to grown, we do more things together, and my husband wants to do them too. We also got our sex back. His interest is the best indicator of my health!"

Jeanette was one of the women who followed the plan I developed in *The Arthritis Relief Diet*, even though she had been on the supplements before I wrote the book. By taking a total dietary approach, she improved even more. From her food diary, Jeanette learned that flare-ups were caused by several foods she liked, such as tomatoes, a few citrus fruits, and several types of meat, especially processed meat. She sticks with her dietary plan and uses the following supplements daily: Vita Lea, B-complex, vitamin C, calcium-magnesium, EPA, Instant Protein, and Daily Fiber Blend. She swears by alfalfa and takes 30 to 40 tablets daily. She is quick to add: "My hair hasn't turned green, and I don't neigh like a horse!"

ALFALFA

Bill's Story

One day I received a long letter from which I quote a section: ". . . on the other hand, the alfalfa has given me considerable relief with the ordinary type arthritis aches and pain. In fact, if I take 15 alfalfa tablets per day along with vitamin C and Vita-Lea, I get complete relief from all arthritis pain within five days, and I can count on it. Then, I can gradually cut down to eight or even as few as six tablets per day and keep the pain under control unless a bad weather front comes through and the weather changes cause my arthritis to flare up. When that happens, a small amount of aspirin alleviates the pain slightly, but alfalfa relieves it completely within five days when I resume taking it."

W. R. A. Jr., M.D.

The author's letter makes a strong case for more research to be conducted, so we can understand the alfalfa experience more clearly. It's important to recognize that Bill learned about alfalfa from a patient, but then by carefully testing himself, he found what worked best for him. You might ask: "Is it in his head?" I don't think so. You see, Bill isn't just another M.D.; he's a board-certified psychiatrist. I think he'd know whether or not it's in his head.

A LITTLE MORE ABOUT ARTHRITIS

In writing *The Arthritis Relief Diet*, I worked with 375 people and personally interviewed nearly 100. Only one woman I interviewed couldn't find any serious stress that preceded her first attack. However, she pointed out that now that the arthritis is established, serious stress will often cause flare-ups. This leads me to believe that environmental factors are so important and deserve special attention.

Environmental factors play an important role in all inflammatory diseases. We usually lump them all into one word: stress. In my opinion, this is an abused word. What we're probably seeing are things that cause changes in hormonal balance. These hormonal balances and other dietary factors change the relative levels of prostaglandins.

A simple way of recognizing the environmental influence on arthritis is to observe how effectively people with arthritis can predict the weather. Although the effect of weather changes on arthritis was laughed at for years, if not centuries, it was finally tested and proven at the University of Wisconsin. They had some people with arthritis live in a phytotron, a large chamber where you can adjust all aspects of weather. Lo and behold, they could accurately detect the changes.

Prostaglandins regulate inflammation. Most drugs, such as aspirin, inhibit the prostaglandin that increases inflammation. EPA increases the prostaglandins that modulate inflammation. The balance of the prostaglandins is influenced indirectly through hormones by environmental factors, including emotional and physical stress. Rheumatoid arthritis is almost non-existent in places such as Greenland, where the natural diet favors a favorable prostaglandin balance.

Recent double-blind studies proved that gold shots were no more effective than a prescription analgesic, which has far fewer side effects.

Diet has become recognized as an adjunct to treatment, especially in the early stages of arthritis. In several clinical studies conducted in the United States and England, swelling and immobility has been significantly reduced by diet. The dietary studies included heavy EPA supplementation. A paper by E. D. Harris, M.D. in the May 1990

New England Journal of Medicine explains this dietary reaction.

IS IT IN THEIR HEADS?

When many people living in diverse areas have the same experience independently, and the experience persists, you can rule out mass hysteria. You need to search for other explanations. I selected Dr. Bill's letter because he is an example of how an inquiring mind got precisely to an effective supplement level. Alfalfa worked for him. Although I don't believe people should be that precise, other doctors have proposed that alfalfa works because it contains a bioflavonoid that resembles a drug used for inflammation. They argue it works because of this resemblance.

I find this "drug" hypothesis hard to accept. In the constant search for effective drugs that the pharmaceutical companies mount, it would have been discovered, patented, and prescribed by now. After all, the elements for commercial exploitation are all there. In addition, the raw material is easily grown in huge quantities, because alfalfa grows all over the world. I favor the idea that the effect is from the alfalfa fiber. This was first proposed to me by Dr. Hal Ashley. Alfalfa fiber is quite unique in its ability to bind bile acids and other materials eliminated through bile. We often fail to remember that the bile duct is an excretory pathway. These bile by-products, called antigens, can cause flare-ups and even worse, keep the flare-up going. So, getting the right fiber should work to reduce flare-ups. After all, alfalfa's ability to bind bile wastes has been thoroughly tested. In addition, the prodigious amounts of alfalfa used by most people are consistent with this hypotheses. In contrast, if we were observing a drug effect, small quantities of alfalfa should be effective.

Once EPA became available, we had a much stronger foundation for supplementation. Indeed, EPA has formed the basis of clinical studies on arthritis and other inflammatory diseases in the United States, the United Kingdom, Japan, and Canada. These studies have all shown that EPA has the ability to restore prostaglandin balance and reduce inflammation. However, a total dietary commitment is better than just taking supplements.

Benefits of other nutritional supplements, such as Vita-Lea and Instant protein, are obvious. The stress of a chronic illness increases nutritional need. A person with a chronic illness, like arthritis, is likely to have a poor diet. The side effects of drugs all increase nutritional need. Drugs used in arthritis treatment increase the need for several nutrients, including vitamins C, E, B-complex, and the minerals zinc and iron. So, it's not surprising that people gain more energy and feel better when using these supplements.

3 Asthma

LAURA'S STORY

"Childhood stopped when I was five," Laura said, then continued. "From then until the age of 30, I didn't have a day without medication and I don't remember a year without at least one hospital stay of a week or more. In addition to that, a good part of my free time was spent in the doctor's office."

In early childhood Laura sneezed alot and had itchy eyes. By the age of five, her problem was diagnosed as asthma. The doctors said she'd probably outgrow this condition, and prescribed a medication, liquid Marax, to help relieve the discomfort associated with it. Once Laura was on this strong medication, she stopped sneezing and she didn't resume sneezing until she was over 30 years old and off the medication.

As Laura approached her teenage years, her doctor changed her prescribed medication from liquid form to pills. It seemed like she was always getting shots, skin tests, and new pills. Most of the medications for asthma have a side effect of being an "upper" or a stimulant that speeds up metabolism. "I was always jittery and hyper from the medication," she said, "and it's hard for me to believe that people take "uppers" on their own."

WHAT IS ASTHMA?

Asthma is a lung ailment that produces wheezing and breathing difficulty and affects 10 million Americans, causing about 4,600 deaths annually. It is a form of an inflammatory disease in which the small tubes in your lungs become inflamed and won't open to let the bad air out. It feels like the reverse; like you can't get any good air in. That's a little ahead of things, so I'll start with the basics.

Think of your lung system as two miniature trees growing upside down in your chest, with your mouth and bronchial tubes as the trunk and large branches. The outer branches get smaller and smaller, just like on a tree. But in place of leaves, the lateral outgrowth from a stem, a bronchiole leads to what looks like a microscopic bubble or balloon, the alveolar, which is bathed by microscopic blood vessels. In the alveolar, blood picks up oxygen and releases the waste gas, carbon dioxide (CO_2). This miraculous exchange all takes place the instant you breathe.

When you have asthma, the microscopic tube that leads to the alveolar becomes inflamed and swells up. As a result of the swelling, you can force air in, but the bad gas, CO_2, won't come out. When CO_2 builds in your blood, a sensor in the back of your brain screams "breathe." If you can't get the bad air out you panic, because it's like smothering. The whole process takes place in just a few minutes. An extreme attack of asthma could cause a person to pass out and die, so it is not something our brain takes lightly. Breathing is the most basic function, and if it is impaired, the body panics.

Now you can see why the doctors' objective is so clear when someone has an asthma attack: get those microscopic branches, the bronchioles, to relax and let the bad air out. Doctors accomplish this by getting the medication into your blood by using pills or shots. Nowadays, doctors also use inhalers that finely mist the medication, so you take it into your lungs with the air you breathe. During an extreme asthma attack, a respirator is used to force the air containing the drug into the lungs. It can be a mighty frightening experience if you're on the receiving end of the treatment, but it surely beats dying.

Asthma, similar to other inflammatory diseases, such as arthritis and psoriasis, remains dormant for various time periods and then can flare up unexpectedly for many reasons. Even though the victim of an asthma attack might be on medication, an intense flare-up can still come on like a bolt of lightening. A flare-up could result in a day of restricted activity with extra medication, a trip to the hospital for an injection, or, if severe enough, a two-week stay in the hospital. Consequently, precautions should be taken to avoid flare-ups. Sometimes, although rarely, a flare-up can bring on death.

The occurence of flare-ups can be traced to many things, including food. For instance, dairy products are high on the list, and other foods, ranging from meat to shell fish, can be identified. Since there are no firm rules on which foods cause a flare-up, one asthmatic's poison can be another's food. You have to test yourself by keeping a careful food-diary so you can identify the foods that aggravate you and then avoid them.

To make it worse, these foods that cause a flare-up don't appear to be food allergies. They're more correctly called *food sensitivities*, which seem to change from time to time. For instance, you might find eggs are okay now, but you could become sensitive to them next year. So although some food sensitivities will not change, some will change. Therefore, you can't let your guard down.

Food sensitivities behave quite differently than allergies. For example, an allergy that shows up as a rash often requires a very small amount of the food. In contrast, one woman I interviewed, who was sensitive to eggs, could get along with eating just one egg. But if she had two eggs on one day or one egg daily for three days, she'd get a flare-up. She is sensitive to eggs, but definitely not allergic to them.

Laura is allergic to shellfish, among other things. Once she inadvertently ate some shellfish and literally went into anaphylactic shock (a hypersensitive reaction). Anaphylactic shock is so severe that you pass out and can die. Thanks to the quick thinking of her doctor, Laura's life, in this case, was saved with an injection of Benadryl to help her body calm down and recover.

Besides food, other things can cause asthma to flare up, such as the hair on pets, fresh paint or varnish, falling leaves, grass, dust, spring pollen, and some things most people don't notice particularly. Sometimes a combination of factors complicates the condition even more. For example, cigarette smoke seems to aggravate asthma. If the asthmatic attack is caused by some other irritant, such as new mown grass, the addition of smoke will make the flare-up a lot worse. In other words, if you react to eggs and eat them inadvertently when people around you are smoking, your attack could be far more severe than if you simply ate some eggs. Think of smoke as the promoter, and eggs as the initiator of a flare-up.

I've interviewed many asthmatics and all of them list stress as a flare-up promoter. Emotional or physical stress is sure to promote an attack and often a trip to the hospital. Emotional stress could be the loss of a loved one, a bad grade in school, your work environment, family problems, and so on. Physical stress, for instance, could be a chill, overexertion, fatigue, eating the wrong food, or exposure to fumes. There are no firm rules.

A COLLEGE FLARE-UP

Laura's husband Scott learned she had asthma while they were dating in college. One beautiful fall day in Indiana, Laura and Scott spent the afternoon walking through the woods around their college campus, rolling in piles of autumn leaves, and talking and conspiring about the future—things young couples have done since time began. Fall colors and young love had invigorated their spirits. By evening, the air was clear and crisp and the sky was filled with bright stars that looked like you could reach out and touch them. In order to get Laura back to her dorm on time, Scott was walking at a rather fast pace, and several times Laura asked him to slow down. Finally, she explained that she had asthma and didn't want to cause a flare-up. This was Scott's first encounter with asthma.

Laura slowed down on the walk home because she knew she had over exerted herself all day and had been exposed to a lot of dust. She didn't want to take any chances. That night in her dormitory room, she paid a high price for her day of fun.

"My lungs couldn't get air. I felt like there was no more air in the room. I was too weak to stand up." She sounded scared just recounting the episode. "Finally, I crawled on my hands and knees down the hall to the next occupied room. It took all my strength to pound on the door."

Our scene shifts now to the hospital where Laura was put on a respirator, a machine that causes your lungs to relax and expand, so medication can be administered directly into your lungs. Medication was used to relax the bronchioles, the microscopic airways, so she could start breathing normally. Scott was called to her bedside and got to see what an asthma attack is all about. After a few days in the hospital, Laura returned to normal.

Normalcy is a subtle problem that plagues all asthmatics. When they're not having a flare-up, they outwardly appear quite normal. Consequently, most people get the impression that asthmatics don't have any illness at all, that it's "in their head," or perhaps they simply have a cold. Since most people never see an asthmatic having a serious flare-up, they have no idea of the seriousness of the disease. Witnessing an asthmatic attack can be a frightening experience.

LOVE CONQUERS ALL

Scott became well acquainted with asthma, but love and biology prevailed, and he and Laura were married. Scott accepted a position in Las Vegas, where Laura also landed a job as the band director at the local school. By this time, Laura was on heavy-duty medication, which included Marax and a Primatene Mist inhaler, among others.

Like many young couples in their age group, they had a water bed. Scott developed a sense for life at sea because Laura, being on asthmatic medication, was always on "uppers." Most folks move a little in their sleep, but Laura was more restless than a tom cat during a full moon when eight local female cats are in heat. "Sleeping on a water bed was like being at sea," Scott laughed. "I actually felt a little woozy at first, then I got my sea legs."

During the eight years they lived in Las Vegas, they were blessed with a little girl, but Laura also had five additional two-to-three week hospital stays for her asthma attacks. That's just about one major stay each year. Trips to the emergency room were too many to count. Scott became quite knowledgeable on what would and wouldn't work for Laura's asthma.

One typical attack would go like this: A flare up would occur and Scott would take Laura to the emergency room. The intern or resident, not having had experience with such a severe case of asthma, would give her about two-to-four shots of epinephrine, because that's what the book said to do. After about two or three hours, she'd be admitted to the hospital where she would stay for a few days or up to three weeks, depending on circumstances.

Laura and Scott learned to give shots of Bricanyl, which relaxes the bronchioles. This would help suppress the attack in its early stages and allow Laura to breathe. This precautionary measure is much like the shots people who are extremely sensitive to bee stings carry with them to help prevent severe shock. Laura and Scott became very good at giving shots and even their daughter became accustomed to her mom getting them.

During these years, life was never normal for anyone in the family. Long work hours, job stress, being a wife and mother, and constantly being "hyped" from medication zapped all Laura's energy; she was forever tired.

After eight years in Las Vegas, Scott accepted an offer for a better job in California, which meant that Laura wouldn't have to work any longer. Since she had become very interested in drugs, this was her opportunity to return to college for an advanced degree in pharmacy. They both were very excited, but didn't look forward to the actual work involved in relocating. Needless to say, the stress of moving accumulated and on moving day, Laura was admitted to the hospital for an eleven-day stay. Friends pitched in to help Scott and fortunately, everything went smoothly.

By the time they moved to California, Laura's condition had worsened and she was now on steroids. Steroids are big-league inflammation fighters. Even though the objective of these drugs is to keep you out of the hospital, living with their side effects is a stiff price to pay. For instance, among the side effects are fluid retention, tiredness, and accelerated bone loss. For Laura, daily naps became routine, just to stay awake. When she asked her doctor how long she'd be on the steroids, his answer was very clear: "For the rest of your life."

Drugs can save lives but have to be used very cautiously. Many asthmatics use a class of drugs known as bronchodilators that relax and expand lung airways during an asthma attack. They are often dispensed in inhalators. Some of the side effects from these drugs are irregular or rapid heartbeat, increased blood pressure, difficulty in urinating, nervousness, and dry mouth.

LAURA FINDS NUTRITION

One especially bad episode turned out to be a blessing in disguise. Laura had an attack that her inhaler didn't stop, so she went to the hospital. The emergency-room physician gave her the wrong medication and made things worse. After a few days in the hospital, she recovered, but during her stay a new acquaintance can to visit her and said, "I think a friend of mine might be able to help you build yourself up. Would you mind if she called you at home?"

Since Laura had tried just about everything else, she agreed. So, when the Shaklee distributor called, she listened. It was a new beginning for Laura's life and the end to her asthma. Three days before she and Scott left to attend an asthma-clinic for couples in Denver, Colorado, Laura started taking Shaklee Vita-Lea and Instant Protein. On the morning they took off for Denver, she felt better and actually enjoyed the long drive from California to the clinic.

The week spent at the clinic was very enlightening. The staff taught them many things about asthma that they didn't know or hadn't learned from experience. One important point they learned was that the drugs used for asthma don't cure the disease, they simply stop the symptoms. In fact, the drugs actually paralyze parts of your lung so you don't sneeze. Laura realized she hadn't sneezed since she was five years old. Almost 30 years ago!

Another side effect of Laura's medication was bone loss. The doctor explained that steroids wash calcium from the bones. This bone loss is especially critical in the pelvic area where it leads to hip replacement in people with asthma or other diseases, because they must use steroids for so many years. The drug is a trade off. You get the miracle, but you pay a price.

During her stay at the clinic, Laura continued taking the Instant Protein and Vita-Lea, and by the end of the week she felt even better. When she returned home and was ready to refill her supplements, she added a few more to her order after listening to a tape her distributor had dropped off. She added vitamin C and 30 alfalfa tablets daily. Although she was skeptical at first, she did notice an improvement. She sneezed! Something must be happening.

Laura added more supplements. She was taking the following: Vita-Lea, alfalfa, Instant Protein, beta carotene, B-Complex, vitamin E, zinc, calcium-magnesium, and a couple Herb-Lax. One constant side effect of the drugs was constipation, but she was now regular.

Two months after she started taking Shaklee products she felt so good, that she asked her doctor to help her eliminate steroids. Working together with him, they started to reduce the steroids slowly. Laura had been asthmatic for 35 years, so a few weeks or months wasn't a long time.

Eliminating steroids was good news. But there was more good news. Once off steroids, Magnetic Resonance Imaging showed her bone loss had started to reverse itself. If it continued, her bone density would be back to normal for her age.

A dark cloud blotted the sunshine of her progress in the form of migraine headaches. Her distributor suggested taking EPA supplements. The migraines left a few days after she started taking the EPA and have never reappeared.

Six months after starting the nutrition program, Laura,

with her doctor's help, was off all medication. For the first time since the age of five, the only pills she took were nutritional supplements. Within a year, her bone density returned to normal for her age, daily naps were no longer necessary, and she had more energy than she could ever remember, even as a child.

Two and a half years have gone by without a single asthma attack. Laura knows she'll always have the disease, so she follows her daily nutrition program faithfully. The good nutrition program keeps the disease in remission, but it will return if she lets her guard down for an instant. If a flare-up occurs, she knows her doctors are there, but she hopes she never needs their assistance again.

As if to prove a point, Laura remarked about a friend who followed a similar nutritional program for her asthma with comparable results. One time her friend's asthma subsided, so she thought she was better and stopped following the plan. Her asthma returned, so she went back on medication. Her friend incorrectly concluded that the nutrition had failed to cure the disease. It hadn't. What she didn't realize was that all nutrition does is help the body keep the remission under control. Nothing cures asthma.

IS IT IN HER HEAD?

No! That doesn't mean that attitude doesn't help, but what Laura experienced is real. Consider the nutrients and the roll they played in Laura's conquest.

Laura was on big-league medication, with all the stress that it brings. In her own words, the drugs are "uppers," cause constipation, and accelerate bone loss. That all adds up to an increased nutritional need for vitamins, minerals, and especially calcium The steroids increase the need for B vitamins.

Instant Protein gives her body the tools it needs for tissue repair. But it does more. It provides additional energy, "staying power" or stamina. Stamina lets you feel as good at the end of a day as at the beginning.

So by starting a good nutrition program, Laura helped her body deal with the constant stress it was under. She met the additional nutrient needs that stress and drugs impose on any body. In addition, alfalfa might have been an unsung hero in this story.

Alfalfa is especially rich in a type of fiber we call saponins. Saponins are especially effective at binding and accelerating removal of the wastes that accumulate in the gall bladder and pass out through the bile duct. These wastes, often called antigens, get recycled if they aren't removed, and constantly aggravate a chronic condition like asthma or arthritis. Alfalfa fiber, and I believe it's specifically the saponins, is effective in eliminating antigens through the stools. Alfalfa is the best known food source of saponins, and the second best source, beans, are less than one-fifth as good.

Although EPA helped the migraines clear up, it also helped the asthma as well. EPA supplements are the most efficient source of the omega-3 oils, which help to modulate inflammation. Hippocrates discovered this in 450 B.C. when he found that flaxseed oil helped reduce asthma attacks. EPA in capsules is more practical than flaxseed oil and keeps better.

Other nutrients helped Laura cope with the stress her body will always need to fight. They include the B-complex of vitamins, vitamin C, and zinc. Vitamin E helped her lungs repair themselves and restored the complex fluid which bathes the alveolar. This fluid, rich in vitamin E, helps neutralize irritants that promote asthma attacks.

It's important to note that Laura and her doctor made a good team and worked together. She didn't quit her medications "cold turkey" on her own. With her doctor's watchful eye, she cut back a little each time until she reached zero. You don't go from over 30 years of taking medication to taking none in one step. In fact, many asthmatics will never get back to zero medication. However, any reduction in medication is a step that will add years to your life and life to your years.

CHAPTER

4 Cancer and Chemotherapy

DELORES' STORY

"Hello, is this Doctor Scala?" After acknowledging the question, I detected an accent in the voice that was definitely of Spanish origin. "Doctor Scala, I have cancer." There was dead silence, so I quickly asked, "How can I help?" There was a slight pause and then the caller said, "A friend told me that you could tell me what supplements to use. I saw you on the "700 Club" and my friend got your address for me. I'm going for surgery on Monday (it was Friday) and the doctor says I'm going to need chemotherapy after the surgery. I'm scared."

When the caller said she was scared, it was an understatement. I could hear the fear in her voice. She only spoke after a long pause; then her voice had a tremble that signified stress. I tried to ease the situation by talking about her family and background.

Delores was 34 years old at the time. She and her husband Antonio, Tony for short, had two girls aged four and six. They had emigrated from Mexico, became citizens, and worked hard. They managed to buy a small house which was the result of a long struggle. Tony was a skilled woodworker and made custom cabinets. Delores worked as a secretary for a company that did business in Mexico. I realized that this family describes the dream that brings people to America: We came for a better life; we worked as laborers to educate our children; our children will become doctors and professionals; our grandchildren can become people of great letters.

Philosophy aside, I realized that Delores needed guidance in the form of nutrition advice and some optimistic support. I recommended some nutritional products that I thought would help her and suggested she find a local Shaklee distributor in the yellow pages. She said she would and also promised to purchase the group of products which included Instant Protein, Vita-Lea, beta-carotene, B-Complex, Daily Fiber Blend, and calcium-magnesium.

Delores started with Instant Protein, Vita-Lea, and calcium-magnesium that Friday evening, and continued taking them until Monday morning when she was admitted to the hospital for a mastectomy. While she was in the hospital, her husband Tony called me. I told him that I wasn't as concerned about the surgery as I was about the chemotherapy. My strategy was for Delores to get in the habit of taking Instant Protein and Vita-Lea each day. I explained to Tony that during chemotherapy Delores would probably lose her sense of taste, so everything she ate would taste chalky and she would also become nauseous. Under those conditions, people tend to avoid food, so it's easier to stick with a simple habit like the one I recommended.

BREAST CANCER: CHEMOTHERAPY

Breast cancer strikes 16 women every hour in the United States, and five women die from it every hour, 24 hours daily, seven days a week. On average, women are 35 when their breast cancer is diagnosed. The cancer probably starts at least five and possibly 20 years before it's big enough to be diagnosed. If detected early enough, no one would die from breast cancer. The reason people die (men also get it) is because the cancer has spread, usually via the lymphatic system, to other organs and tissues in the body by the time it's diagnosed. It usually spreads via the lymphatic system to other organs and tissues.

A surgeon has two options: a mastectomy, total breast removal, if the cancer is not localized; or a lumpectomy if the cancer is small and definitely localized. During surgery, the surgeon usually removes some lymph nodes from under the arm for a pathologist to analyze. If any lymph nodes have cancer, the usual course is chemotherapy.

Chemotherapy employs highly toxic chemicals that kill rapidly reproducing cells. The principal involved is simple. Cancer cells are the most rapid growing cells in the body. Therefore, if you give the body a poison that kills dividing cells, statistics dictate that it has a better than average chance of killing a cancer cell. Experts admit that there ought be a better way, but there isn't at this time.

However, for chemotherapy to succeed, it requires from eight to twelve weeks of treatment. Chemotherapy varies according to the cancer, but is usually done twice a week. In this way, the laws of probability give a high chance of killing any residual cancer cells. Since cells enter the period of division at different times, the idea is to keep the chemotherapy up long enough to get them all until the body cannot tolerate the process any longer.

If you get the idea that chemotherapy is not an exact science, you're correct. The more rapid the cancer is growing, the lower the chances of success. To make matters worse, some cancers are more resistant to chemotherapy than others.

Chemotherapy also hurts the body's cells. In short, it gets some of the good guys along with bad guys. People lose their taste because taste-bud cells don't reproduce under chemotherapy. The same with hair follicles, so your hair falls out. Side effects from chemotherapy include severe nausea, liver damage, and other problems. Chemotherapy is a very grim process to go through, but it's all we have at this time. Experts all agree that many other better techniques are on the way. Someday we will probably see chemotherapy as a barbaric treatment.

About 69 percent of women who had breast cancer, and either go for chemotherapy or radiation, survive. That's a good success rate compared to lung cancer, for example, where about 11 percent survive; or liver cancer, where only about 5 percent survive. Cancer is considered cured if the victim survives five years.

DELORES CONTINUES

"Surgery was the easy part," Delores said, over the phone. She went on, "Three out of ten lymph nodes were positive. My doctor wanted me to start chemotherapy as soon as I'm well enough. Do you think I should?"

Delores' question hit me like a knife. Somehow, Delores had to make that decision with Tony and her doctor. I simply told her to ask her doctor what he felt her chances for success would be. She screwed up all her courage, took Tony with her, and asked her doctor. He told her that about 85 percent of women with her type of cancer and lymph involvement make it through the five-year period after chemotherapy.

When Delores told me what her doctor had said, I then asked her how many things she starts have an 85-percent success rate. She decided to go the chemotherapy route.

Delores lost her hair and her taste went out the window. She never got nauseated and, in spite of her hair loss, she felt good through most of the chemotherapy. She returned to work and her co-workers couldn't believe her optimism. She never wavered from taking Instant Protein, Vita-Lea, and calcium, but she did put the other supplements on the shelf from time to time until she was through with the chemotherapy.

I would talk with either Tony or Delores every few days. The family was doing quite well under the circumstances; in fact, the children were being real troopers. Both Delores and Tony became depressed occasionally, but Delores had her moments of real despondency.

How did Delores do? Let me tell you in her words. "I told my doctor I was going to stay with the supplements. He said it was okay with him. About half way through the chemotherapy he asked me if I would mind talking with other women who didn't want to take chemotherapy. I asked him what I could say to them? After all, I didn't speak good English. Well, the doctor said he was so impressed by the way I came through the chemotherapy, that he wanted me to share it with others and reassure them that it's worth while."

From that point, the story gets better. Delores slowly increased her supplement program; in fact, the entire family did. She completed the chemotherapy course. The doctor plans chemotherapy again in six to twelve months. His strategy is to stop any other cancer that may have survived, before it gets started again.

HARRIET'S STORY

Harriet found a lump on her breast one morning while showering. "I checked it about six times that day because I couldn't believe it. If wishful thinking or checking it every few hours could get rid of a lump, mine would have gone." Harriet went to the doctor; he called for a biopsy which turned out to be positive.

"I decided on a lumpectomy and the surgeon agreed. The tumor looked localized and he said that if my lymph nodes were negative, he would stay with that strategy. He said that after surgery I would have radiation therapy."

Harriet was a Shaklee user and asked me if there were any special supplements she should use. I told her that what she was doing was fine, but to add more beta-carotene, about five a day, all the way through the radiation. I also urged her to continue taking her 400 or more International Units of vitamin E.

RADIATION

Radiation therapy has a similar approach to cancer as chemotherapy does. High energy X-rays are targeted at the tissue surrounding the area where the tumor was removed. The object is to kill cells that are rapidly dividing (i.e., cancer cells).

Beta carotene is a natural chemical that nature uses to protect important tissues and cell components from radiation. It won't stop the X-rays from hitting the cancer cells, but it modulates them enough that there's minimal tissue damage around the target. For example, in the skin cells where beta carotene goes, it will help prevent radiation burns. But if an X-ray hits a cancer cell, the cancer cell dies.

BACK TO HARRIET

"I'm turning into a little orange," she said jokingly. I told her not to worry; it just meant she was getting enough beta-carotene. She had already discussed this observation with the radiologist and she, too, said it was all right.

Depression and irritability are normal by-products of radiation therapy. Harriet had both. However, at her examination when she was well into the radiation, the radiologist commented that she didn't show any significant signs of radiation burns. She came through the radiation with flying colors. Now Harriet has a mammogram every six months and an annual examination by her doctor. She is considered cured.

A recent analysis of breast cancer survivors brings

many factors to the fore. Unfortunately, being financially poor reduces your chances of survival. It's probably because going through the welfare system means a longer time is required for diagnosis and treatment. But nutrition is also an important factor. Better nutrition favors survival. So, not only does good nutrition help these women through chemotherapy, but an independent study says it helps their bodies deal better with the cancer itself.

COLON CANCER

Phil's Story

"I couldn't believe the doctor when he said he saw something with the sigmoidoscope and occult blood test that he didn't like during my annual physical," Phil said, and went on to describe his ordeal. "Within two days I was in the hospital for a colonoscopy, biopsy, and, if appropriate, surgery. My wife Jane is a nurse and wouldn't let me put it off another minute. I could barely tell the people at work. I'll never forget how scared I was. It was like drowning. My whole life kept passing in front of me."

Colon Cancer

Actually Phil had colorectal cancer, because it was in both his colon and rectum. At age 42, he was young for this type of cancer, because the average age of diagnosis is 52. He was one of the 17 people every hour in the United States who are diagnosed with colorectal cancer. Fortunately, he was not one of the seven who die from it every hour in the United States. By the way, that's every hour, 24 hours a day, seven days a week. Cancer doesn't take time off.

Cancer in the large intestine usually begins as a polyp which looks like a small wart. Polyps turn cancerous at a rate of about 2 percent in the first five years, and then double every few years after. Consequently, about 24 percent are cancerous after 20 years.

Look at the statistics like this: If a hundred people aged 35 lined up, and each one of them had at least one polyp, two of them would have cancer in five years, eight in 10 years, and twenty-four in 20 years. What's bad about intestinal polyps is that you don't feel them. Therefore, the objective of an annual physical is to spot a polyp before it becomes cancerous. The occult blood test is given to detect any polyp that is advanced. By the age of 50, most of us will have at least one polyp.

Back To Phil

"I woke up with my wife at my side. She didn't mince words when she told me I would always have a colostomy. At first I wanted to cry, but then I realized that I was alive and that was the first step."

Phil went home and, with his wife's help, learned how to clean his colostomy. He had to irrigate it daily for about an hour to an hour and a half. He used this time to read and has become one of the most widely read people I know. He stuck with his Shaklee program while he was in the hospital and at home preparing for chemotherapy.

"I thought the chemotherapy would be hell. In fact, I was almost going to say 'no' to it, but after reading up on the procedure, I decided the odds were in my favor. I set up a supplement program that made sense to my wife and me, and my doctor didn't object. I used Instant Protein, Vita-Lea, B-Complex, vitamins E and C, and zinc. My doctor told me not to use B-Complex or Vita-Lea when I got chemotherapy. He said one would interfere with the other."

Phil took the doctors advice. He came through the chemotherapy with flying colors. In fact, his doctor personally called me and said he took chemotherapy without any of the major side effects. Indeed, Phil didn't lose his sense of taste, didn't become nauseated, and kept working throughout the chemotherapy.

Since he was just about bald before the chemotherapy, he's not sure if he lost any hair or not. Phil's nutrition program carried him through the entire ordeal. He healed quickly from the surgery and came through chemotherapy with optimism. He regulates the flow through his colostomy by using Daily Fiber Blend and is in excellent health.

WHAT'S IN THEIR HEADS

None of these people, and the many others I could have chosen from, came through their ordeals by either wishful thinking or some placebo effect. Each person went through surgery well, recovered quickly, and had an equally healthy experience in either chemotherapy or radiation.

It's hard for me to think of a more difficult experience than to face cancer head on and win. Worse yet is to survive the surgery, face chemotherapy, and then go through it knowing that it's a systematic process to poison your cells with some of the most toxic substances known.

I can't think of a time in life when super nutrition is more necessary. Your body is hurting; you can't absorb nutrients as well as you did; you lose your appetite; toxins are flowing through your veins; and you're scared to death. Words like stress don't come close to describing what's going on.

There's no hope of eating a balanced diet during surgery and chemotherapy. Besides, who can tell you what a balanced diet is for someone under those conditions? How do you get enough of the healing nutrients? I believe there's really one answer: super supplementation!

PREVENTION

Cancer can be prevented. Prevention calls for lots of cereal, fruits, vegetables, and moderate exercise. Specific preventive nutrients are vitamins C, E, folic acid, and niacin. The minerals selenium and calcium are also essential. Probably the most widely known preventer is beta carotene, but factors in the cruciferous vegetables rank a close second.

Regularity from fiber is essential to prevention. We need 30 grams of fiber daily and only get about 12 grams. The lack of regularity shows up in many forms of cancer, although it's especially germane to polyp formation.

I urge everyone to purchase a copy of *Prescription For Longevity* (Pub. E. P. Dutton), which will be released in March 1992. This book discusses prevention in detail.

CHAPTER

5 Cholesterol

TOM'S STORY

"I noticed that I would get a pain at the base of the front of my neck when I played a hard game of tennis. Since I was in good condition, I just thought it was aging; after all, I had just turned 50. One day while playing tennis with a doctor friend, I got the same pain, so I asked him what he thought it was. He asked me if I had noticed any congestion or indigestion, and since I hadn't, he advised stopping tennis and exercise, in general, until the cause of the pain was determined. He told me to come by his office so he could take some tests.

About 10 days later the doctor gave Tom an EKG, took blood tests, and listened to his heart from every imaginable angle. After reviewing the test results, he recommended Tom to see a cardiologist and have an angiogram.

In preparation for the angiogram, the cardiologist reviewed Tom's EKG and blood work which showed his cholesterol level at 325. Tom was overweight, though not seriously, but he had carried this extra weight for many years. The cardiologist scheduled him for an angiogram, a technique in which the doctor can see any clogging in an artery or vein around the heart. In searching the arteries around the heart, a long catheter, or tube, is inserted into either a large vein in a leg or arm. A skilled cardiologist works the catheter up to the area near the heart. During this procedure the patient is x-rayed, which allows the doctor to see how the catheter is progressing on a video. Once the catheter is in the correct position, the surgeon releases a dye that shows up on the screen, because it's opaque to the low energy X-rays. He can then watch the dye enter and leave the cardiovascular arteries and the heart on video, and record it to play back as often as necessary.

An angiogram permits the cardiologist to decide how clogged or occluded the various arteries are around the heart. In addition, the surgeon can assess any damage done by a heart attack. Angiograms are slowly being replaced by other techniques which use ultrasound and other methods. However, when Tom was being analyzed, an angiogram was the only method available.

BACK TO TOM

"I had prepared myself for the worst, but it was worse than I expected. The doctor wanted to schedule me for a quadruple bypass at the first opening. I told him I'd like to try diet and exercise. He said I wouldn't live long enough to reverse the damage. Three of my arteries were about 90 percent occluded, and another one was about 75 percent occluded. He said I was lucky I hadn't had a heart attack."

Tom had the bypass. He didn't like it, but by the time he got home, he realized he could breathe better. The hospital had an exercise and diet program for bypass patients, so Tom joined. His wife Margo went to the classes with him.

BYPASS SURGERY

A bypass is a miracle-made routine. As its name implies, it is a surgical technique in which a partially clogged artery leading into or away from the heart is bypassed by a piece of vein usually taken from the patient's leg. Although it has become routine, bypass surgery is deep-chest surgery and is very, very serious. Usually it's performed after the patient has had a heart attack. In a post heart-attack patient, bypass surgery is much more serious, because the risk of an attack during the procedure hangs over the operating room. However, less than 10 percent of patients die from the surgery. All things considered, that's an impressive record. Tom was fortunate that an alert doctor discovered his situation before he had a heart attack.

BACK TO TOM

Bypass surgery is almost routine in many large hospitals. While Tom's chest was opened up, the surgeon decided on a fifth bypass, so Tom's quadruple bypass became a quintuple bypass. Post-operative recovery wasn't fun for Tom, but it was normal by medical standards. In spite of clogged arteries, he was in good physical shape. His heart was strong and there was plenty of collateral circulation. In a strange way, Tom's circulation was better after surgery than it had been ten or more years previously.

"In a few days I could tell that it took less energy to do things. Sure, I ached from my scars, my legs hurt from where they took the veins, but I could still do things with less effort. I guess I had grown accustomed to working with only partial circulation." Tom tells it as if it were yesterday.

Three years later, his doctor jolted his attention. Again, Tom tells it clearly. "My doctor asked me if I wanted another bypass. I looked at him as if he was joking. Then he told me it was no joke. My cholesterol had gone up to 300. Looking back, I realize that I let my job dictate my life. My exercise had dropped to almost zero. I had breakfast meetings at least twice a week, lunch out everyday, and dinner at least three out of five evenings in restaurants. Although I usually ordered fish or pasta, the sauces were there, wine with most meals, and face it, I had added a few pounds." Tom tells it as if he was blaming himself, but his experience is typical.

GOOD NEWS: BAD NEWS ABOUT BYPASS

Most people who have bypass surgery are candidates for a second round in five years. This happens because bypass surgery corrects a problem, but it doesn't do anything about the cause.

Tom had everything against him. Sounds strange, but think about it. He had an aggressive personality, a high-tech sales job, was on the road 30 percent of the time, and his dinner and other meetings were routine. Besides all that, he had lots of internal stress with his drive to constantly improve his performance.

In addition to his lifestyle, Tom is also representative of many people. His cholesterol and triglycerides have a tendency to elevate. His body probably doesn't make enough HDL cholesterol (good cholesterol), or his body lacks the ability to remove the LDL-cholesterol (bad cholesterol).

Tom's dietary intentions were good, but the road to hell is paved with good intentions. Cholesterol and triglycerides are mostly dietary-fiber and dietary-fat problems with excess calories, often from sugar or alcohol, thrown in. Taking care of the fiber usually helps to bring the others into line.

BACK TO TOM

"I was embarrassed. If the doctors objective was to scare me, he succeeded. I told him I'd get on the diet right away and start exercising. He said he'd give me three months and then he'd like to try medication. It was a new challenge for me," Tom said, with his blue eyes flushing with excitement.

"My wife had told her friend where she works about my problem. Her friend sold Shaklee products and agreed to speak with me about a new product they had for lowering cholesterol. I figured I had nothing to lose and everything to gain." He laughed as he recalled that evening.

"I spent $175 after seeing a short video and scanning a book on cholesterol by Bruce Miller. Margot and I went home with Fiber Plan, Vita-Lea, EPA, vitamin C, Instant Protein, and Meal Shakes. If cost and success were proportional, I'd be a winner."

Tom worked Shaklee into his life. He used Fiber Plan at each meal as directed and a fourth of a serving at night, because it made him feel full. Meal Shakes were substitute meals to help him lose weight when he was on the road or eating in his office. He didn't like Instant Protein, but Margot made him take it in the morning when he didn't eat.

"In three months, I had my follow-up visit. I had my blood taken a week before so it was on the doctor's desk when I walked in. The doctor looked at me and asked me what I had been doing, then he showed me my results. My cholesterol had dropped from 300 to 235 in three months!" Tom tells it like he was bragging about a new child. "Not only that, my HDL cholesterol had gone up from 43 to 55 and my triglycerides were down from 300 to 200. My doctor was happier than I was." Tom was in his element; he had competed and won, but it wasn't enough.

He agreed to have blood tests taken every three months. The follow-up test three months later came in with a cholesterol reading of 200, and three months after that, it was 190. His HDL cholesterol remained between 50 and 55. Tom's triglycerides have dropped and have remained at 150.

WHAT WENT ON HERE?

Tom, like many men and women, let his health slip away. Diet for him was a series of good intentions. He'd order chicken or fish, eat some salad, and think that was enough. Well, it's not.

Fiber Plan is formulated with dietary fiber that is especially good at binding the bile acids and dietary cholesterol. It binds them tight enough to remove them from the body in the stools.

An average adult requires from 30 to 45 grams of fiber daily. On average, we get less than 13 grams daily. In short, we don't come within a country mile of what we need. So, people like Tom must either change their diet beyond what is practical for them, or add back the missing fiber. That's what Fiber Plan does. Simple, isn't it?

We still need a meal to provide protein, calories, some pleasure, and nutrients. Our food contains about 6 grams of fiber per 1,000 calories. So, to get the minimum, you'd have to eat 3,000 calories daily. Unfortunately, if we ate that many calories daily, we'd all be fat, except for a very small minority.

Most women get along being a tad overweight on less than 2,000 calories, and most men, also a tad overweight, on less than 2,500 calories. Therefore, we get a little less than half the fiber we require. So we've got to add it back, and we can't do it just once in awhile. We've got to do it every day of every year.

Two other parts of this story are often overlooked: they are the HDL cholesterol and the triglycerides. You want the HDL cholesterol to increase and the triglycerides to decrease. Fiber helps accomplish this, but another supplemental oil, EPA, gives them a boost.

Once more, our diet is the problem. EPA is an omega-3 oil and our only meaningful dietary source is fish. Unfortunately, Americans don't eat much fish — less than half an ounce, on average, daily. We add injury to this insult by eating an excess of competing oils from grains that are added to the animal fat we get from meat, dairy, and poultry products and baked goods. So, increasing omega-3 oils calls for either dramatic dietary changes, which are close to impossible for all but a few, or using EPA supplements. In my opinion, it is foolish not to accept the products of our technology to improve our health and prevent illness. Supplements are an outcome of our technology that enables us to make up our dietary shortfalls.

TOM'S PLAN

Tom continues his supplement plan, Fiber Plan with meals, and three EPA capsules daily. His cholesterol has settled in at about 190, with his HDL averaging 50, and his triglycerides are lower, nearing 150. He's probably more healthy than he was 20 years ago. He also exercises by jogging. Tennis is fine, but it's seldom regular enough or consistent.

His use of the Meal Shake to keep his weight in line is practical. He has added Daily Fiber Blend to help his regularity. Also, during this time he has become a user of other supplements, including Vita-Lea, vitamin C, vitamin E, and sometimes B-complex. He describes his use of B-complex this way: "I seem to relax better when I use it. My doctor says I should relax more."

RUTH AND JIM

Ruth and Jim decided that the best way to share a good thing was to make it a group effort. They rounded up 15 friends and asked a direct question: "Who wants to improve their health?" All hands went up. "All you've got to do is purchase this product, Fiber Plan, and take it with each meal. No other changes, just do whatever you're doing. To start, you'll need to have a blood test for cholesterol and then again after six weeks." Everyone stuck to the plan and followed the directions.

Ruth is a former high-school science teacher and likes to compile numbers. She wasn't interested in what people said happened, she wanted to see the results. Her experiment produced the following results:

Average Blood Cholesterol Change in Six Weeks

Before	After	Total Drop	Percent
244	220	24	11%

This tells a good story. For example, a cholesterol of 244 is a moderate risk for heart disease for someone 50 years or older, but a high risk for heart disease for someone 35 or younger. Therefore, she brought the older members into a low risk, but the younger members were moved into a moderate risk. Some individual numbers prove a point.

Five Individual Results
Six-Week Change in Cholesterol

Before	After	Drop	Percent
260	234	26	10%
256	224	36	12%
146	116	30	20%
389	339	50	13%
228	191	37	16%

Five of Ruth's volunteers illustrate two points which are especially instructive: all of them got positive results, and their health improved. So, her proposition was fulfilled.

The person with the lowest starting cholesterol (146) got excellent results. She proved that no matter how good your health is, it can still improve.

The person with the highest cholesterol level, 389, moved his risk in the right direction. His next measurement, after another six weeks, produced a similar reduction, and now, almost a year later, he is within easy distance of 200.

Unfortunately, not everyone sticks closely with a program, and Ruth pointed out what I already knew. "Some people admitted that they didn't stick with the original plan. They only took the Fiber Plan twice a day and often skipped some days." But, that's real life for you. I'm delighted because everyone got good results and a few of them got spectacular results.

IS IT EVER TOO LATE?

One problem in the United States is that we are bombarded with information. To sell articles, a journalist only needs to wait awhile and an expert will emerge with a contrary position. It didn't take long for experts to come out and say that they don't know if Fiber Plan helps older people, say over 55 or 60, to lower cholesterol. They went on to say, "why should we try to get cholesterol down, if we don't know if it helps?"

Hogwash! The experts could have said: "It's bound to help, but we don't know by how much. In fact, we aren't sure how to measure the good that it does. We only know that high cholesterol shortens life and doesn't lengthen life. So there's much to gain and nothing to lose."

6 Chronic Fatigue Syndrome / Epstein-Barr Virus

BECKY'S STORY

"Did you ever feel tired when you awoke from a good night's sleep? I did." Becky spent her sixteenth year always being tired. As Becky says, "I would come home from school, go to my room, and lay down for a minute. Next thing I knew, Mom was calling me for dinner, and I'd have to force myself to get up and eat. I would make it through dinner, an hour or two of homework, and then drop. This same routine would start all over again the next morning.

Close friends would tell me how tired I looked. They were right. I always had bags under my eyes and my complexion seemed dull. My hair even lost its luster. I often felt depressed and that there was no use to anything.

About every six-weeks I would go to the doctor. First our family doctor thought I had mononucleosis. He took a blood test that came out negative. Then he decided my tiredness was caused by a thyroid problem, so he ordered more tests. Nothing showed up. Next I saw an endocrinologist and she tested me for a number of things. She began with the thyroid, glucose tolerance, and went to other glands, but could find nothing. A gynecologist examined my female organs and they turned out to be fine. Finally, we just stopped going to doctors because it was getting no where. They had done test after test and kept calling for more tests. If tests could have solved the problem, I would have been cured.

My mom read about the Epstein-Barr virus and decided I should be tested. This test turned out to be negative, too. It proved nothing for the hundredth time. All I wanted to do was sleep, and I always woke up tired.

My school work suffered, not because I couldn't get the work, but because I was in a fog from being so tired, and it took all my energy to concentrate. All I wanted to do was rest. Gym class, which met three days a week, was the worst. A session of calisthenics left me totally exhausted. When I started to fall asleep in school, Mom decided my problem was really serious; it wasn't that I was just going through adolescence.

Finally our family doctor had me see a psychologist. It was the last straw when she started asking me about boys and sex. I was so tired that the last thing on my mind was boys or sex. I simply refused to see her anymore.

I started losing my friends because I didn't have the stamina to do anything outside of school work. I stopped going to athletic events and other social activities, simply because I was too tired.

My mother was beside herself with worry. She spoke to anyone who would listen. Sometimes it was embarrassing, like the time she asked a shoe salesman. One day she spoke to a Shaklee distributor. This lady gave her a short write-up on a woman who had recovered from Chronic

Fatigue Syndrome. Mom decided to put me on the same nutrition program. I was willing to try anything, so I figured a few vitamins couldn't hurt.

Mornings became a nutrition ritual in our house: Instant Protein, Vita-Lea, B-Complex, vitamin C, and calcium-magnesium. The Shaklee lady had told my mother the magnesium was important. I didn't need my monthly periods anymore in order to get bloated. The Instant Protein did it for me quite effectively.

After about a month, the bloating from the protein had gone. In retrospect, I should have started with a smaller amount. I actually started to like the stuff and affectionately called it my 'morning mulch.' Although I didn't realize it at the time, I stayed after school a few times with friends. Then, about a month after I started on my mulch program, I went to a basketball game. It was fun and I even went out for hamburgers with the kids afterward.

By spring, I was doing things with my friends after school. I asked a boy to the Sadie Hawkin's dance and got invited to the spring hop. My social life started coming back. Sure, I liked to sleep in on Saturday and Sunday mornings like everyone else, but I wasn't waking up tired any longer.

We never did figure out what I had. Our family doctor says he's seen these symptoms in a number of people — mostly women or teenage girls. He said the medical experts call it *Chronic Fatigue Syndrome* (CFS). They think it's caused by a virus. Unfortunately, there's no cure; it just takes time to leave your system.

I believe him when he says there's no known cause or cure, but my experience says nutrition helps you get better sooner. Shortly after Mom started me on the program, I could feel my strength returning. Sure, it didn't happen overnight, or even in a month, but I got a little better every day. I only wish I had started my nutrition program sooner."

WHAT'S GOING ON HERE?

Chronic Fatigue Syndrome is officially recognized as a disease. It has been identified in teenagers and adults of all ages. A study at the Washington University School of Medicine found that there was no clear link with any known virus. The most widely known viruses tested were the Epstein-Barr virus and coxsackieviruses. Chronic Fatigue Syndrome seems to develop after an acute illness such as the flu. However, CFS can appear several months after the flu is gone.

Chronic Fatigue Syndrome is a malaise-inducing illness in which the most common symptom is a lack of refreshing sleep. Teenagers in the Washington study got six to twelve hours of sleep and woke up tired. Exercise caused them to have extreme fatigue. Becky described both symptoms clearly. A secondary symptom is depression and a feeling of uselessness. Sound familiar?

Along with chronic fatigue, symptoms vary and include headaches, an inability to concentrate, just like Becky experienced, sore throats, nausea, and even vomiting. Typically, a teenager with CFS will miss an average of 34 days of school in a six-month period. Some teenagers in the Washington study missed 80 days in six months!

BARBARA'S STORY

"I have always been full of energy. I'm a grandmother three times now and run my own color and image business. One spring, just over a year ago, I started waking up with headaches in the back of my head. The winter that year had been particularly damp, and I picked up a good case of the flu like many other people in our area, but I recovered from it more quickly than most of my friends.

What began as headaches when I awoke, led to an upset stomach before an hour had passed. Neither the headaches nor nausea persisted more than a few hours and wouldn't come every day, but they would leave me worn out. I began to realize that I was always tired. Things I did on a regular basis became a serious chore.

I was accustomed to working all day at my business and relaxing in the evening with my husband. We have an indoor pool and our recreation routine included a swim before dinner to get our heads clear. I would always feel refreshed after my swim. I found myself going upstairs to change into my bathing suit and just falling asleep on the bed. The bed was like a siren calling me. My husband Bill would have to wake me up and I'd usually skip the swim with the excuse that I would just go and make dinner. Then I'd forget to make dinner or just sit in a chair and watch the news on television.

I began to lose my concentration during the day. In my business I speak to a lot of people, mostly women. A few times I found myself forgetting their names in the middle of a conversation. Worse yet, my mind would drift and I'd forget what we were talking about.

Now and then, I would try to go to bed early, about 9:30 p.m., thinking I'd wake up in the morning feeling refreshed. Somehow, I thought that all I needed was a good night's sleep. After sleeping like a log for about ten hours, I'd still get up feeling tired. If it wasn't for my husband, our business would have failed. He carried the ball.

I began to look around for something that would help me. Doctors usually remind me of my age and would talk about slowing down; or they'd say it was a postmenopausal malaise, whatever that meant. One doctor did a thyroid test, but the results were negative. Every doctor took a blood test. Sometimes I think they believed that testing would cure the disease. Finally, I listened to a friend selling vitamins. She was full of energy, so I figured, if I could get half of her energy, I'd be okay.

I started on Vita-Lea, Instant Protein, B-Complex, Herb-Lax, and a few other supplements, including Liqui-Lea. Bill bought $181 worth of supplements that very evening. Starting the next morning, he made me take one or two of them every day. I gagged on the protein the first time, and was told to start with one-third of the amount I was taking. Within a month, I stopped having the headaches and started swimming again. I didn't climb out of the pool exhausted. In fact, just climbing out of the pool was a step forward. Within two months I was waking up with some energy. People started asking me what I had done, because I had so much energy. They said I looked relaxed.

Before that, I couldn't get myself looking good. I had to use more make-up and add conditioners to my hair to give it body. Good friends said I looked tired. They would comment that I was working too hard and that we should take a vacation. Little did they know that I was sleeping more than they were.

Now, a year later, I realize I had what is called *Chronic*

Fatigue Syndrome. I also understand how the nutrition program helped my body fight it off and rebuild itself. I've read up on this disease and concluded that each expert has their own opinion. Some say it's magnesium, but my magnesium tests were always normal. I don't believe that anyone really knows what causes or cures this disease. In fact, I believe that our body does the curing, if it gets the right nutrients. I also believe that anyone who hasn't had the disease, has no idea of what it's like. That includes the doctors. Unless you've felt the "bone-deep" tiredness that takes all your strength, you don't know what it is to be really tired. It doesn't compare to being tired from a hard workout or from plain hard work. It's worse than being tired from caring for children or grandchildren or even the tiredness I experienced when my mom died. There's a character to the tiredness that defies description. You have to experience it to understand the despair it brings."

IT'S IN THEIR HEADS

Chronic Fatigue Syndrome is a real disease. Most experts believe it results from a virus, but they don't know how. The most likely viral candidate is the Epstein-Barr virus. In fact, CFS has also been called the Epstein-Barr Syndrome. However, some people with CFS don't test positive for the Epstein-Barr virus and some people who test positive for it don't have CFS. If this sounds confusing, it is, and probably will be for some time to come.

When someone has CFS, they can't seem to become rested; they're always tired. You could say this is a mental or at least a partially mental condition. However, a mental component doesn't make it any less real. It just makes it more difficult for science to attack. The fact that victims of this disease feel completely exhausted after exercise, proves it's not mental; and that they feel tired after a good sleep, proves that it has a mental component. The headaches, nausea, and lack of concentration also confirm this.

Nutrition definitely helps in two ways: it gives short-term energy, and provides the tools for the body to re-build. Both people in these two cases got more energy and stamina when they used Instant Protein. Instant Protein contains two sources of energy: one is carbohydrates, and the other is derived from the non-essential amino acids it supplies. Besides short-term energy, the body needs to re-build whatever system or systems have gone awry. Building anything in the body requires protein, energy, and nutrients. So, it's not surprising that the victims felt better, looked better, and seemed to maintain consistent recovery once they started a complete nutrition program. Since B-Complex seems to help, it suggests that metabolism is involved.

Reports of recovery times required for CFS range from one year to five years. These time periods imply that the body must restore itself. Self healing is always a slow proposition. In short, the recovery time is not like an infection that an antibiotic can knock out in a couple of weeks; or a malfunction in an organ, like high blood pressure, that can be corrected with medication. Nutrition makes a big difference, and nutrition is always slow-motion medicine. That's why time is so important.

7 Crohn's Disease (Inflammatory Bowel Disease)

HANNAH'S STORY

"Mother told me I had a rectal fissure when I was two years old. My first recollection of rectal bleeding was when I was 10 years old and in the fifth grade. By junior high school, I was missing a lot of school because of vague, but severe abdominal pains. I just didn't feel good. My parents and the doctors believed me, but the doctors couldn't find anything wrong."

Hannah is an achiever. The day she was inducted into the National Honor Society, she was at home sick. She had been tested many times for ulcers and mononucleosis, but the doctor was unable to make a diagnosis. "Tired" could have been her middle name, even though she performed so well in school.

By her senior year in high school, Hannah was vomiting almost daily. At five foot two inches and 70 pounds, a doctor today would have suspected anorexia or at least chronic malnutrition, while he searched for a chronic digestive problem. Being a national honor student while all this was going on, tells you a lot about Hannah's spirit. She finished high school without her illness being diagnosed, aside from some vague hints at psychosomatic problems.

College was tough; not because of the school work, but because of her illness. Her problem, still undiagnosed, went regularly from constipation to diarrhea with rectal bleeding. Nausea and vomiting had become routine for her. By her sophomore year, chronic fatigue had her falling asleep sitting-up in class. Somehow she managed to keep her studies up. She was finally hospitalized and a definite diagnosis was made.

"You've got Crohn's disease," the doctor announced. "In 1962, that diagnosis was so rare, that most doctors weren't even familiar with the disease," she said. "In 1962, Crohn's disease was only 28 years old as a recognized bowel disorder. I was almost that old," Hannah added.

CROHN'S DISEASE

Crohn's disease is an inflammatory autoimmune disease affecting the small intestine. If an inflammatory bowel disease strikes the large intestine, it's named according to the colon. For example, colitis or ulcerative colitis strikes the colon. A person can have both, such as Crohn's colitis. Crohn's colitis means the inflammatory disease involves both the small and large intestines, usually where the two meet.

Nowadays, these diseases are lumped under the heading Inflammatory Bowel Disease or IBD, for short. The cause of IBD is not understood. About 35 percent is hereditary, and the rest is felt to involve childhood viral infections, possibly a bacterial infection, and other environmental factors. However, the disease may not show up until many years after the infection. IBDs are characterized by flare-ups, which usually include devastating diarrhea and, as Hannah said, rectal bleeding. Flare-ups are often stress related, good and bad stress, but stress doesn't cause the disease. It's only a precipitating factor.

Studies by psychologists have shown that people with IBD do not have common personality traits. These studies support the notion that personality or mental characteristics are not causative factors. However, once established, stress is a clear factor in causing flare-ups.

Autoimmune means that the immune system attacks the body's own tissues at specific sites. For example, in rheumatoid arthritis, the immune system attacks membranes in the joints — say the hands. The body reacts with both inflammation and rapid growth in the area. So, in rheumatoid arthritis, the joints become inflamed and distorted by excess growth. Similarly with psoriasis, to name two relatively common examples.

In Crohn's disease, an inflamed small intestine can become totally blocked, or the opening can shrink to the size of a drinking straw or smaller. Eating under those conditions leads to nausea and vomiting. But it gets worse. Malabsorption and lactose intolerance almost always accompany Crohn's disease. This means that you don't absorb nutrients from food and must avoid dairy products. In our society, dairy products are the source of some important nutrients.

If malabsorption and an inflamed intestine aren't bad enough, the autoimmune aspect makes it even worse. In Crohn's disease or colitis, the body attacks inflamed parts of the intestine. In these areas, the intestine becomes scarred where the attack occurs. These scars are commonly called strictures. Think of the knurled, deformed hand joints of some arthritis victims. A somewhat similar condition occurs in the intestines.

Moving from the small intestine and Crohn's disease to the large intestine and colitis, think of ulcers developing. These ulcers produce bleeding and intense pain. Needless to say, seeing blood in your stools is always a scary experience.

Physicians have several approaches: steroids to stop the inflammation in an acute attack; drugs to quiet the intestine in a mild attack; and surgery to remove the diseased portions. Surgery often leaves the victim with an artificial opening for eliminating stools. This opening is usually an internal pouch that usually requires emptying four or five times daily. Though difficult, the pouch usually provides a better life than living with the chronic, aggressive diarrhea. Sometimes the opening is a simple colostomy, such as Phil had from his cancer.

Flare-ups characterize all inflammatory diseases, especially inflammatory bowel disease. The disease can remain dormant, in remission, usually for months and then flare up with a vengeance. At these times, the best approach is to quiet things down. This is done with drugs, rest, and sometimes hospitalization with complete feeding by total parenteral nutrition, TPN. This feeding is accomplished by entering a large vein, usually in the chest, and using a nutrient solution to feed the patient.

Recently, inflammatory diseases have been experimentally treated with EPA and the by-products of its metabolism, the leukotrienes. This approach, at the frontier of science, holds out much hope for the IBD victim. In addition, up to ten successful intestinal transplants have been done at one medical school. Transplants are the last resort, but sometimes the only solution.

I recommend my book entitled *Eating Right For A Bad Gut*, which deals more extensively with the dietary and nutritional aspects of IBD. With this background information, let's get back to Hannah's story and those of two other people.

One negative side-effect of IBD is an increased rate of colorectal cancer. The rate for IBD patients is about 216 times that of the normal population. This rate can be reduced 50 percent by taking folic-acid supplements or a complete supplement that contains folic acid. This is an excellent example of the preventive power of nutrition.

HANNAH'S STORY CONTINUED

In 1962, the concept of lactose intolerance in IBD was unknown. "My doctor recommended milk shakes to build me up." But in spite of that advice, Hannah did well in school and married her college sweetheart. Her marriage is an example of good stress. The day after her wedding, Hannah's Crohn's disease flared up. "I was in extreme pain. Doctors tried cortisone injections to stop the inflammation." She continued, "I had to live with my parents and my husband Allan visited me on weekends, because he had a job some distance away." Hannah and her husband had to build their marriage under extreme stress.

We know, in hindsight, that Hannah's doctor had good intentions with the milk-shake advice, even if it was bad food for her. Milk shakes probably kept the inflammation going. Then add the stress of a wedding (recall that good or bad stress is still stress), and Hannah was set up for a severe attack. At least it held back until the morning after her wedding.

Hannah's post-wedding Crohn's flare-up didn't subside and the doctors recommended surgery. She put it off for a few weeks and visualized herself coming out of surgery cured. Read the afterword of this book for some reflection on the important, positive aspect of visualization on health. Hannah went under deep surgery to remove the diseased parts of her intestine.

After surgery, the doctor said, "Hannah, it was localized in three places and we got it all." Finally, Hannah and Allan could start a normal life. Normal, except for occasional impactions from her intestine being closed by strictures from the surgery, and the chronic fatigue from malnutrition.

Strictures, or scar tissue, often develop after Crohn's surgery. These localized areas are where the intestine healed after surgery. Strictures are places where undigested food can lodge and literally stop things from moving down the intestine; an impaction develops.

Overcoming rectal impaction from strictures near her rectum caused secondary problems. The only solution was to stretch the scar tissue by rectal dilations. This office procedure was very painful, but necessary.

When Crohn's disease was in the early stages of recognition and doctors had little experience treating the disease, they advised against having children. That has all changed now, but at the time, Hannah and Allan decided to adopt two girls. Adopting children is often said to be a sure way to become pregnant, and that's exactly what happened to Hannah.

Hannah managed to deliver a healthy daughter during

this stressful time in her life. Weekly rectal dilations continued for six years. You might be wondering, if scar tissue is the problem, why not just remove it? Not so easy. At that time, the doctor reasoned that more scar tissue would form. He was correct. Scar tissue on the intestine is much more complicated than on another part of the body. So, as painful and stressful as the dilations were, it was the most reasonable approach.

In the late 1970s, Hannah developed other problems. One was cystic breast disease, which some doctors blamed on the steroids she was given. This is not necessarily correct and the jury is still out. Chronic fatigue was a constant companion, and she seemed to have acquired allergies. All this time she was unable to put on much weight. Although some women would view this weight problem as a positive outcome, it's not that way in Crohn's disease.

Not being able to gain weight and having chronic fatigue is frightening. People who have these problems must always worry about their health. Add to this, fibrocystic breast disease and the stress of weekly doctor visits, and you can see why Hannah would have been a very scared person.

In 1979, her life changed. She found Shaklee. "My doctors had never believed in supplements. I had tried various store brands, but I couldn't tolerate them. Boy, what a pleasant surprise I got from Shaklee products." She continued to talk about her results. "My energy returned. I gained time because I stopped taking daily naps and didn't have to go to bed so early at night. I gained weight, so I knew I was utilizing my food better. Then, after a few months, the cysts in my breasts cleared up," she said with a sigh.

Hannah gained a new lease on life. Though surgery had cleared the Crohn's disease, she was still sick. Her supplement program took care of that. Within a few months of starting her Shaklee supplement program, she stopped the rectal dilations and has had no problems with strictures since then.

A four-year follow-up examination showed that the stricture in her rectum was gone. With the exception of the diseased areas of her intestine that had been surgically removed, she was normal.

Hannah's diet improved with the supplements. Folks with Crohn's disease usually lean toward highly processed food. Most processed food doesn't contain fiber or any chunks that can irritate the intestine. But unfortunately, eating this type of food carries a price: poor nutrition, including a lack of dietary fiber, unless the processed food is a high-fiber cereal. Her diet now emphasizes the principals of low fat, good quality protein, and dietary fiber, which she gets from fiber wafers. In addition to that, she takes Instant Protein.

Hannah faithfully uses Shaklee products. Her daily supplement plan, which she takes four times daily, includes Vita-Lea, alfalfa, B-Complex, calcium-magnesium, zinc, Vita-C, vitamin E, Instant Protein, EPA, beta carotene, and fiber. At bedtime she takes one Herb-Lax.

WHY?

Hannah's experience with Crohn's disease—years of intestinal problems and fatigue, with her illness undiagnosed—is typical for the time period involved. During those years, the number of digestive-system specialists was relatively small, and her family doctor was simply not trained to handle this type of specialized problem. Therefore, Hannah's chances of seeing a doctor experienced in diagnosing Crohn's disease were somewhat remote. Fortunately, she met up with a physician who made an effective diagnosis. Her successful surgery confirms his findings. She was lucky because her disease was mild enough so that she was left with a normal rectum after surgery.

Once Hannah found Shaklee, her health fell into an excellent pattern. People with Crohn's disease usually have malabsorption. The only practical way to overcome malabsorption is by taking more nutrients. A further complication in her case was the surgical removal of significant portions of her small intestine, which reduces the nutrient absorption area. This removal capacity makes it more difficult to get adequate nutrients from food. It is a second reason for using supplements.

An even more difficult obstacle to good nutrition is when the lower part of the small intestine and the initial part of the large intestine are surgically removed. This removal compromises the body's ability to extract several B vitamins and the mineral zinc, and also jeopardizes water balance.

Hannah is one of a large number of women who have cystic breast disease and get relief from vitamin E. About 16 percent of women with cystic breasts will get total relief from vitamin E; their cysts will completely disappear. About 80 percent will get some degree of relief, even if it's only relief from irritation and minor clearing of the cysts. In this regard, Hannah is, indeed, fortunate to be part of the top 16 percent.

The clearing of Hannah's scar tissue and the complete

healing of the fissures, which dogged her after surgery, are testimonies to good nutrition. You can't ascribe Hannah's healing to a single nutrient, because several nutrients were involved: zinc, vitamin E, vitamin C, and several B vitamins. Also, protein is essential in the healing process. Therefore, supplemental protein is important. It's important to note that people with Crohn's disease are more likely *not* to get enough zinc because of malabsorption.

Hannah's IBD was corrected with surgery, but she has maintained her health with good nutrition. Let me introduce you to a person with IBD who has been able to manage without surgery and the support of Shaklee products.

BOB'S STORY

Ulcerative Colitis

Like many people, including Hannah, Bob has food sensitivities and thinks of them as allergies. It's best to determine these food sensitivities by keeping an accurate food-diary. Bob is sensitive to tea, spinach, and dairy products. Any one of these foods causes a flare-up that usually lasts for two weeks.

Stress also causes Bob's flare-ups. Although it has been proven that stress does not cause IBD, it's definitely a factor in the flare-ups. As Bob put it, "Several doctors said stress didn't cause my colitis, but experience tells me that it causes flare-ups. A flare-up is preceded by a brown fluid oozing from my rectum for up to two weeks. When the flare-up starts, pain, bleeding, and diarrhea come like a freight train. I take Azulfadine and stay on it daily for up to two months."

Bob learned, by experimenting on himself, that Shaklee products help minimize the number and intensity of flare-ups. These products include Vita-Lea, vitamins C and E, alfalfa, Fiber Blend, EPA, beta carotene, calcium, and B-Complex. Notice how similar Bob's supplement program is to Hannah's.

MARLENE

Crohn's Disease

Unlike Hannah, Marlene has had extensive surgery for her Crohn's disease, which is still active. She is representative of a serious dilemma: After surgery, Marlene was left with only 10 feet of a normally 13-foot small intestine. Her large intestine was completely removed, which necessitated an internal pouch that must be emptied through its opening in her side, five times daily. She continues to have flare-ups, which doctors fear may call for removal of still more of her small intestine. A very grim prospect. She's thin and has a lot of trouble keeping her weight up.

Marlene takes nine tablets of four different medications daily and several others during periods of flare-ups. Her supplement use is similar to Hannah's and Bob's, although her level of each supplement is not the same. She regularly uses Vita-Lea, vitamins C and E, iron, alfalfa, calcium, and B-Complex. So far, this program has kept her healthy.

MRS. O

Crohn's Colitis

Mrs. O has similarly experienced the role of stress in her flare-ups. She has kept an excellent food-diary and found a number of foods that unequivocally cause flare-ups. For example, beets or beet juice, and milk will cause violent attacks. Other foods which cause normal flare-ups, if they can be called normal, are chocolate, melon, citrus fruit, and grapes.

Mrs. O identified a definite seasonal influence on her disease when she said, "All my attacks occur in the spring. What do you think of this seasonal influence?" I followed up and interviewed more people who identified spring and fall as the seasons in which their flare-ups were most likely to occur. Seasonal changes are consistent with the inflammatory nature of these intestinal diseases. Spring and fall are times of large changes in the barometric pressure in most parts of the United States. Barometric pressure has been proven a factor in both rheumatoid arthritis and migraine headache, two other inflammatory illnesses, so it's safe to include IBD.

Mrs. O uses Shaklee products. Her program is almost a duplicate of Hannah's, so I won't go into any further detail. She has been able to avoid surgery for her Crohn's colitis. Surgical removal of some benign polyps and hemorrhoids was necessary. She has also had lithotripsy for kidney stones. Often kidney stones are a side effect of colitis because of medications and water balance.

I'd like to quote Mrs. O because she summarized IBD so nicely. "Shaklee alfalfa tablets made a dramatic improvement in my bleeding problem. Doctors are surprised when they examine my colon, because it doesn't show any permanent damage. The ulcers have consistently healed clearly. I believe the Shaklee products, especially beta carotene, help prevent my attacks. It's also good for people with Crohn's to take more vacations to relieve any stress."

WHY ALFALFA?

Both alfalfa and Fiber Blend show up with special mention by people who have IBD. Why? In *Eating Right For A Bad Gut*, I discuss both the need for fiber, especially soft fiber, and the need to avoid the fiber matrix. Both of these products, alfalfa and Fiber Blend, provide excellent fiber without a fiber matrix. Other fiber supplements have the soft fiber, usually from psyllium husks, but they don't contain hard fiber without the matrix. To get enough fiber from alfalfa tablets, you need to use about 30 tablets a day, which only amounts to about a tenth of an ounce. However, such a prodigious number of tablets often scare many people.

8 Cystic Breast Disease

HANNAH AND JANET

"I could feel a change within one week." Janet was ecstatic. She had been diagnosed as having cystic breast disease, which is characterized by small cysts in the breast. These cysts have a consistency like grains of sand, which cause the breasts to feel irritated, and hurt. As Janet said, "It's scary, because all you think of is cancer. Even if the doctor says it's not cancer, you can't get it out of your head."

Janet was introduced to Shaklee products when she attended a lecture on nutrition. After hearing that vitamin E could help her cyst problem, she started taking two 400-I.U.s of vitamin-E capsules daily. Within one week the irritation disappeared and she felt as if the cysts had diminished. At the end of the first month they were almost gone. When I spoke to her about six months later, the cysts were completely gone.

Besides taking vitamin E, Janet also took other preventive measures. She drank no caffeine-containing beverages, such as coffee, tea, and soft drinks, and took Vita-Lea, Instant Protein, and other Shaklee products. However, she attributes her success to vitamin E.

HANNAH

Hannah was put on steroids off and on during her episodes with Crohn's disease. She believes these steroids had some influence on the development of cystic breasts. Since she was having so much trouble with Crohn's disease, and the doctors had assured her the cysts were benign, she didn't worry about them.

When Hannah started on Shaklee products, she took about 1,200 I.U.s of vitamin E along with other products. This amount of vitamin E is about twice the level used in clinical studies on cystic breast disease.

Almost in passing, she said, "The cysts in my breasts disappeared." Cystic breasts were obviously not a major concern for her, but they are gone.

WHAT DOES SCIENCE SAY?

In my book *Prescription For Longevity*, I discuss cystic breast disease and vitamin E in more detail. Briefly, about 80 percent of women who have cystic breast disease will experience relief of irritation from using vitamin E. About 16 percent will see complete disappearance of the cysts, and up to 40 percent will experience partial clearing.

Other dietary factors that help reduce breast cysts are

the elimination of caffeine and other stimulants. Smoking seems to also aggravate cysts. "Stop smoking" is good advice for anyone, but it's especially important for these women.

Clinical studies have proven that vitamin E used as a supplement is safe up to 3,000 I.U. daily. So, the 600 I.U.s used in cystic breast disease, though high by RDA standards, are well within the safety limits.

9 Detoxification

MIKE'S STORY

"I worked a lot with Agent Orange in Vietnam. Sure, the instructions said not to get it on your body or your clothes, but there wasn't any protective clothing around." Mike continued, "The instructions also said to wash your clothes immediately after working with Agent Orange and shower thoroughly. You work with the stuff and it wasn't always possible to shower. Heck, we'd just go eat. We'd usually go several days between showers and got accustomed to wearing the same work clothes for several days before we could get them washed." He laughed. "Heck, we were young, it was Vietnam, and we were happy to be alive."

During that time Mike recalls getting a serious rash around his joints. "It was like bad case of prickly heat and I'd get it severely on my elbows or under my arms. But," as Mike put it, "you show me someone who has been in the army or marines who didn't get a rash." I can't argue with Mike's logic. Most people who do a tour of military duty get at least one rash. Given the heat and humidity in Vietnam, a rash was a common occurrence.

People often ask me about toxins in the body. Even though the concept of toxins in the body is probably as old as our ability to reason, it's difficult to be specific when answering these questions. In the human body, a major function of the gall bladder, kidneys, and intestinal tract is the removal of wastes. It is known that if some wastes accumulate, they can soon cause illness and later death. Even research has shown that women who are chronically constipated are more likely to get breast cancer. Some experts suspect that breast cancer results from the by-products of estrogen metabolism. Therefore, it seems conceptually realistic that bowel regularity helps rid the body of these by-products. Detoxification seems like a good word to describe this elimination.

Animal studies with deadly toxins, such as the carbolines, food dyes, and other materials, support the concept of detoxification. For example, in animal studies pioneered by Dr. Benjamin Ershoff of the University of Southern California, noxious materials were either fed or injected into the peritoneal cavity of these animals. Following these injections, the animals could be detoxified by diuretics, laxatives, and dietary fiber.

A third line of detoxification evidence comes from methods used in many hospitals and clinics all over the world. Dialysis, a procedure that keeps thousands of people alive in the United States alone, is a process that takes over for the kidneys and removes toxins from the blood. Consider the process of chelation, which is routinely used to trap toxic metals, such as lead, mercury, and aluminum in the blood, so they can be removed either by dialysis or the kidneys.

Detoxification is a process that is both necessary and clinically valuable, yet discussions about it are often perplexing. People speak vaguely of rashes and wastes and are too indecisive and unspecific to be helpful scientifically. However, when I came across Mike's story, I could put things together and they all made sense. Mike's story deals with several issues that I hope you find as interesting as I did. First, I need to give you a little more background information.

AGENT ORANGE

Agent Orange is a very powerful herbicide that was used in large quantities by our armed forces in Vietnam to defoliate the leaves from large areas of jungle vegetation. Military experts believed that by clearing foliage, the Vietcong could not hide from our planes. In my opinion, a defoliant constitutes one aspect of chemical warfare, even if the chemical wasn't directly applied to people. If Agent Orange inadvertently destroyed the enemy's crops, it was clearly chemical warfare, because it deprived noncombatants of food.

United States' troops who serviced apparatus on the planes that sprayed the herbicide, came in contact with Agent Orange. Whether or not they used correct safety precautions to prevent personal contact is not an issue here. Many of them routinely came in contact with Agent Orange accidently because of inadequate safety gear, carelessness, sloppiness, or just because there was a lot of it around. Many of these men had health troubles after the war and a large number of them developed unusual symptoms, including cancer. Their children had an abnormal number of birth defects. Although statistics are hard to find, enough people had these problems to attract attention. A general's son who had worked with Agent Orange, developed cancer from which he died. The general was so racked with guilt, that he devoted his life to fighting the system to get funds to compensate these afflicted veterans.

Debate continues over whether or not these diverse symptoms and deaths were caused by Agent Orange. Some experts argue that Agent Orange was not unequivocally proven to be the cause, even though the circumstantial evidence is compelling. Statistical analysis, as it often does, leaves room for further searching and doesn't give a definite end to the debate.

One study that impressed me compared military dogs used in the Korean War to those used in the Vietnam War. This study left no doubt that the Vietnam dogs suffered from more cancer and other chemically-caused illnesses than the Korean dogs. Perhaps, in a world where the politics of human clinical studies are so strong, and statistical analyses are so equivocal, these animal findings will be our best evidence.

With that as background, allow me to tell you a very touching story about detoxification. It brings out the plight of many Vietnam veterans who had contact with Agent Orange and puts the stories you've heard into the lives of two real American people and their families. Mike's story about detoxification is one of the most optimistic Shaklee stories I have ever heard.

BACK TO MIKE

After the army, Mike put his education to work and became an employee of the state social-services system. After a few years in that position, he answered a calling to enter the ministry. Mike became a preacher. Anyone who has heard Mike speak, quickly spots two characteristics: Mike is devoutly religious and has an ability to make himself understood without being overbearing. Consequently, his calling to the Lord's work benefits many people.

Mike retained most of the weight he had gained while in the service and decided it was time to go on a diet. "I followed Dr. Atkin's diet because everyone was using it at the time and it seemed to have a lot of promise. I found it easy to count my carbohydrates every day and still eat the things I liked. I lost 70 pounds and looked great." Mike was close to his youthful "fighting" weight, but the only fight that took place was inside his body.

"I started having headaches that would hang on for several days. The headaches weren't bad enough to put me in bed, but I never felt right. They were always there. I started noticing a bad taste in my mouth. It was a sort of foul taste like I just woke up and hadn't brushed my teeth. The taste lingered. I could drink something like a soft drink and the taste would clear, but in an hour it was back again. When the blackouts started, I got scared." Mike described his illness with a detachment, as if he was describing someone else. His ministry is one of total optimism, so he naturally tends to see a bright side to everything.

While the headaches, blackouts, and foul taste dominated his senses, the rash from Vietnam came back. It was like prickly heat multiplied a hundred times and it wouldn't stop. The skin around every joint was especially

bad. The rash got so terrible under his arms and on his elbows, that the skin cracked and oozed blood. His clothes
would take on a red tinge around the elbow, arm pit, and
knee areas. Only one course of action was available to
him.

Mike went into a Veteran's Administration (VA)
Hospital. When the doctors realized how bad he was, they
admitted him and kept him for a full month. Test after test
was taken and many of them Mike didn't even know existed. The doctors couldn't find any specific illness. This
made things even worse, because medicine is based on
specifics. One doctor worked with Agent Orange vets and
told Mike that the excess fat he carried around on his body
was loaded with Agent Orange. The doctors reasoned that
by losing so much weight, he put large amounts of Agent
Orange into his blood all at once and it overloaded his system. A lot of systems just went awry. For example, he
was tasting Agent Orange. The doctors reasoned that the
Dr. Atkin's diet caused his blood sugar problem.

Mike's blood sugar was so high that the doctors tried
insulin, even though his pancreas was working. The insulin only made things worse, so they dropped that approach. Bringing his blood sugar down didn't stop either
the headaches or blackouts, as the doctors had hoped for.
Mike's response to their well-intentioned tests probably
led the doctors to take the Agent Orange hypothesis more
seriously.

Two things the VA doctors thought they could control
were a chronic staph infection and the rashes. Wrong on
both counts. Antibiotics knocked the staph down, but not
out. Creams and ointments, if anything, made the rash
worse. Mike was one sick man and he didn't respond to
the doctors' treatment at all.

Doctors in the VA hospital admitted defeat with Mike's case and proposed a very generous, alternate approach: "We'll bring you into the VA hospital system as a long-term patient. You'll receive all pay and allowances according to your permanent discharge rank. This will provide you and your family with an income. We'll send you to Walter Reed Army Hospital where you'll receive the expert care and attention you require." There was nothing else they could do.

This generous gesture to help a man, who was desperately ill, is testimony to the VA medical system. The doctors added one more thought to help Mike see things their way: "You're only 35. We don't believe you'll live to see 40 at the rate you're going."

Mike couldn't give up his ministry, nor could he leave his wife and four children. His wife Debby followed the controversy over Agent Orange in the newspapers, magazines, and on television. She decided that nutrition would help solve Mike's problem. She knew he had to get his weight down, so she tried various diets, all based on good nutrition.

All of the diets produced the same result. "As soon as I started losing weight, the blackouts, rash, foul taste, headaches, and nausea started with a vengeance." I don't want you to get the idea that Mike and the family ate poorly. Debby had done a thorough job. They ate good, wholesome food. Even a dietician couldn't find fault with their menus.

Mike's health problems started about seven years after he was discharged from Vietnam. During that time they had three girls and a boy. Mike joked: "Don't feel sorry for my son. The girls loved him because he was the baby and the only boy. He had it made." During this time Mike had gone from the state social services to a ministry in Florida and then on to another ministry in North Carolina where he had grown up. He conducted his ministry with a constant headache, a lingering rash, and occasional blackouts.

If all this wasn't enough, he had a mild heart attack. What he thought was more indigestion, VA doctors determined was a heart attack. Although it was mild, he was left with some scar tissue. The doctors also concluded that he had developed a heart valve problem. All he could do was live with it as best he could.

Most people would say, "lose weight and these problems will clear up." He tried that, but the headaches, foul taste, blackouts, and chronic rash all came back ferociously. He was used to the headaches, but the other problems were unbearable, so he just went along with things.

Mike had been to a clinic in Chicago and was getting ready to drive up again for intensive treatment. Debby had been after him to take nutrition more seriously, so she gave him a tape to play while driving to the clinic. "I don't remember who spoke on the tape. It was a woman who sounded so convincing about good nutrition, that I made a U-turn and went back to the house. I told Debby that we'll make nutrition work."

Doctors in the Chicago clinic were understanding when he called and cancelled. They told Mike to return to the VA hospital and have blood tests taken so they could monitor his progress correctly. Mike recognized the wisdom of this advice, so the next morning he checked into the VA hospital as an outpatient for complete blood work.

Mike's blood work didn't paint a very nice picture. His blood sugar was 510 against a normal of about 110;

cholesterol was 298 against a normal of 180 for his age; and his triglycerides were 490 against a high normal of 150. The results didn't place him at "death's door," but he wasn't very far away. With his physical data, resting pulse of 95, and blood pressure of 150 over 110, he had to accept the "grim reaper" as a close companion.

Debby had a great plan for him. It included a balanced, low-calorie diet, and Shaklee products. "I dove into those Shaklee products with determination," Mike said, and continued. "I took lots of everything: Vita-Lea, Vita-C, Vita-E, Zinc, Formula I, and lots of B-Complex. I had a serving of Instant Protein three times a day; that was my meals. I took eight Herb-Lax every day. If five were enough for an average person, I figured eight would just do it for me." Mike also used garlic and an acidophilus supplement which the doctor had recommended previously.

"I didn't feel better all the time. I noticed a cycle. Every three days I'd wake up feeling great: no headache, lots of energy, no foul taste, and the air felt clean in my lungs. On the other days, I still felt poor and had the foul taste. In about three weeks this cycle stopped and I felt good all the time. I noticed the rash was getting smaller." Mike continued the program, which included taking lots of supplements.

In this early period, the cracked skin under his arms and around his elbows cleared. Everyone he met commented on how good he looked. After the first month, as agreed, he reported to the VA hospital for his blood work.

His resting pulse was 65 and blood pressure was 122 over 72. A new, young doctor was on duty at the hospital and had Mike's folder open as he looked at his one-month blood chemistries: cholesterol 143, triglycerides 152, blood sugar 160. The doctor suspected mistakes had been made, possibly even a mix-up of blood samples.

"Would you stay overnight and let me repeat your blood work?" A diplomatic way of him saying that there had been a mistake; these results were flukes. Mike agreed. He was feeling good and was confident his results weren't a fluke in the system. The new doctor took his blood and sent it to a private lab for faster analysis. The second analysis confirmed the first month's results. All the numbers were within analytical tolerances. The results were solid.

Mike says, "I could see excitement in the eyes of the doctor. He had a special interest in Agent Orange cases and wanted to follow my case. Every month was the same. The young doctor became so excited, that he would almost jump for joy with the results." Unfortunately, this doctor was transferred and Mike didn't see him again.

After six months, Mike was 62 pounds lighter and weighed 235 pounds. Even for a big man, 235 pounds is still big. His total cholesterol was 132 and his HDL cholesterol was 48. This yields a risk ratio of less than three, which is excellent at any age. Triglycerides of 86, yielding an LDL cholesterol index of 67, is good even for a teenager! A blood sugar of 154 was the lowest it had ever been in his entire life. Mike was the picture of health. Physical data included a resting pulse of 62 and blood pressure of 110 over 65. The staph infection was gone, and each other test from the blood analysis was comfortably within normal range.

VA doctors posed another request. "In view of your history and the mild heart attack, we'd like to do a stress test followed by an echocardiograph." An echocardiograph is a way of looking at a heart with sound waves. In the hands of an expert, an echocardiograph is like watching a heart work as if it was in a glass case, open to view. Mike agreed to both tests. He was on a crusade to prove that good nutrition could defeat any health problem.

His stress test on the treadmill was excellent. He got his heart rate to 189 against his maximum of 195. He couldn't quite reach the maximum in the time allocated. After the normal cool-down period, his vital signs, heart rate, blood pressure, and so on, returned to normal within ten minutes, just as it should.

Next came the echocardiograph. It showed a normal working heart and only an experienced expert could spot the slight scar left by his heart attack. The doctors summarized Mike's progress in two simply beautiful words: "You're healthy!"

In view of Mike's progress and continued program, the doctors followed up in another six months. Dull. Everything was normal to excellent. He had lost more weight and was getting close to his 200-pound target. He had added years to his life and life to his years.

Mike continues following his Shaklee program of Instant Protein, Vita-Lea, B-Complex, and the other supplements. He now takes Herb-Lax more moderately when he needs to, and no longer tells Herb-Lax jokes when he speaks. Mike is just a normal, gifted man who spreads God's word through his ministry.

MIKE'S DAUGHTER

Elizabeth's Story

"We always called Elizabeth our little 'spice of life,' " Mike said. "She sang in church even before she could read the words, was the perennial optimist, and friendly to everyone." Elizabeth has smooth, Irish skin with freckles. Her red hair would make her look like a native on any Belfast street. When Elizabeth became quiet and stopped smiling, Debby and Mike became concerned. Since all children have ups and downs, they didn't worry until she started walking funny. She kind of slouched her shoulders. Later, when her ordeal was over, her parents asked her why she didn't tell them she hurt. Her reply was logical: "Dad, with all your troubles and going to hospitals, I just couldn't give you another problem."

In reviewing Elizabeth's condition, a doctor and chiropractor came to the same conclusion: "It's a stage she's in and she'll just grow out of it." So Mike and Debby went along with their conclusions until one night when Elizabeth couldn't climb out of a bathtub. This wasn't any "stage" for a six-year-old.

Trips to local doctors turned up a big nothing. But "chance favors the mind that's prepared," and by chance, a medical missionary friend of Mike's was passing through town. She examined Elizabeth and believed she felt an abnormal growth on her spine. She told Mike and Debby to get her to a bone specialist quickly.

A bone specialist examined Elizabeth's spine and put her in the hospital that very day. The doctor said, "It's not negotiable, she goes in now!" The orthopedic specialist called on a pediatrician and oncologist for support. They strongly suspected cancer. After some debate with the pediatrician, Elizabeth was transferred to another hospital attached to a medical school where the doctors had more experience with childhood cancer. Little Elizabeth was put in a ward for terminal cases.

Elizabeth was given a CAT scan that showed the tumor was extensive and had injured her fifth vertebrate. Subsequently, she was put to sleep for the tumor surgery which lasted three hours. Mike and Debby waited for the verdict. Both the neurologist and oncologist had long faces when they came into the waiting room. "We've sent a biopsy to the lab and want to prepare you for the worst. It doesn't look good, but we'll know tomorrow morning after the pathologists examine the biopsy."

That night Mike prayed for the Lord to be quick with Elizabeth. He asked for her suffering to stop. At nine in the morning, the doctors came into her room beaming, "It's not malignant." Mike knelt down and prayed thanks to the Lord right there with a room full of people. He also prayed for the doctors.

Elizabeth didn't need any chemotherapy or radiation. The doctors wanted her to go home, rest, and try to rebuild her strength. What remained of the tumor would localize and surgery could be postponed for several years, at least. At worst, after more surgery, they felt Elizabeth might require a brace because of the bad vertebrate. But one step at a time, and getting her strength back was the present plan.

"We put Elizabeth on so much beta carotene her skin turned orange. We gave her calcium-magnesium and even Vita-Cal in hopes her bones would make up their loss from the tumor." Besides taking calcium and beta carotene, she also took the normal supplements.

At the first month follow-up, the doctors were delighted with Elizabeth's progress. Her back muscles were lining up nicely and she was generally healthy; the second follow-up visit was set for three months later.

At the next follow-up visit, a new doctor examined her, because the original attending physician took a new position in a Wisconsin hospital. After a routine examination, he had Elizabeth touch her toes so he could examine the tone of each vertebra by hand, one at a time. He looked at Mike and asked, "Which one was the problem? Was it five or seven?" The doctor couldn't tell if either one had been bad. That was all Mike needed to hear. She was cured!

What happened after that visit is history. Elizabeth's spine cleared up completely. The doctor has no plans for surgery and sees no need for braces. An annual checkup is necessary as a normal, routine procedure. Elizabeth is on the books as "cured."

IS IT IN MIKE'S HEAD?

No, of course not. Mike's story is typical of men, especially those who were overweight, worked with Agent Orange, and didn't take enough precautions. Some were much worse than Mike. In contrast, other men who worked with Agent Orange had no reaction at all. Mike's weight worked against him. So long as he put weight on, the Agent Orange had a reservoir for itself and didn't spill out into his blood. His downfall was the first diet he followed, the Atkin's diet, that mobilizes fat very rapidly, because it causes a precipitative drop in carbohydrate reserves.

A low-carbohydrate diet forces the body to burn fat rapidly. With most of us that's the desired result, but for Mike, this type of diet released lots of the toxin into his blood. The doctor had it right the first time when he suspected the Atkin's diet of causing his blood sugar problem and releasing the Agent Orange from his fat deposits. The doctors were also correct when they said a low-carbohydrate diet is hard on the pancreas. That particular type of diet definitely belongs in a skillful doctor's hands.

When Mike followed a good diet with lots of protein and nutrients, he was helping keep his metabolism normal. The Herb-Lax and fiber helped rid his system of all the toxins that were also probably getting into his intestines through his gall bladder.

Mike's three day cycle of feeling poor, then great, is not surprising, as it probably related to the use of carbohydrate reserves with water loss. Rebuilding these reserves takes about three days while fat is burned. Once he reduced his body fat content and achieved a higher lean-body-mass ratio, he got rid of the Agent Orange. From then on, the toxin was gone and his body was normal. His blood chemistry and physical signs proved this point.

ELIZABETH'S CASE

In contrast to Mike's story, Elizabeth's story is speculative. There is circumstantial evidence that children of Agent Orange victims have had a higher portion of tumors and bone problems. Only extensive research will ever get to the bottom of the controversy, but there's a lot of support.

Elizabeth's tumor and related spinal problem could have been a defect resulting from Mike's exposure to Agent Orange. Recent research has shown that some birth defects are often traced to the sperm. In the past, the assumption was made that these problems came through the ovary of the mother. The facts say otherwise. Statistical analysis shows that environmental factors, such as Agent Orange, are the causes. It's reasonable that it took six years for the tumor to reach a size that could effect Elizabeth's spine. The slow growth-rate of the tumor is also consistent with other findings.

Mike and Elizabeth's success came from good nutrition coupled with good medical care. Debby deserves recognition for providing a good basic diet. Good diet, supplemented with Shaklee products, gave each body the support it needed to rebuild.

A few research papers have shown that beta carotene helps to shrink tumors. Some experts have shown that the body produces a very small amount of retinoic acid from the beta carotene. They then speculated that retinoic acid is responsible for the tumor shrinkage. Obviously, more research is required for a definitive answer. For now, chalk up one more observation that favors super nutrition.

CHAPTER

10 Eczema: Psoriasis

JOSHUA'S STORY

Joshua's mother Pam told me her son's story, which began when he was three-years-old. I'll describe the salient events of what happened, and how Joshua became a normal boy.

Pam's daughter, Kerry, who is about nine years older than Joshua, broke out in a serious rash after receiving her standard immunizations for school, and had to be hospitalized. The doctor thought Kerry had an allergic response to the shots, because the rash, covering about half her body, developed in a few days and lasted just over two weeks. The rash was treated topically and cleared up, so when she was released from the hospital, Kerry's skin had returned to normal. The doctors concluded that she had had an unusual reaction to her immunization shots and they let it go at that. Kerry has never been troubled again.

When Joshua was born he seemed to be troubled with mild, but persistent skin rashes off and on. Recalling Kerry's problem, Pam decided to hold off Joshua's immunizations as long as possible. However, as a three-and-a-half-year-old, he was ready for preschool, and since the system says, "Thou shall have shots," Pam reluctantly went ahead with the immunizations. In her words: "You can't really fight the system and stay sane." Shortly after the shots, she and her husband took a Shaklee cruise as part of their award for having built a business. While they were away, Joshua stayed with his grandparents. During that time, his grandparents noticed that he had been itching and digging at his skin during the night. They were disturbed, because every morning he would wake up covered with scratches and cuts.

When Pam returned, she realized something was seriously wrong. To say Joshua was "scratching and digging" was the understatement of the year. He looked like he had been trying to referee cat fights. Pam immediately took him to see the doctor. Joshua's problem was diagnosed as eczema, an inflammation of the skin which is characterized by redness, edema, oozing, crusting, scaling, and itching. Scratching or rubbing can lead to other problems, such as an infection, that starts when dirt gets into a cut. Eczema is a description of what's going on, but it's not the cause.

The skin is the body's largest organ. It's about 20 percent of the body's weight and has the largest area exposed to all elements. The lungs actually have a larger surface area, but their environmental exposure is both restricted and controlled by the fluid with which their surface is bathed. Besides, the lungs have a system to remove many materials in the air before they get into the lungs, so the skin is the largest freely-exposed organ.

Our skin is a unique organ because it has many functions of its own, but it is greatly influenced by what is going on in the rest of the body. You might observe from personal experience, that when your stomach is upset, your facial color might go from pale white to sickly green. Or if you eat the wrong food, you might develop a rash or "blotches" over various parts of your body that can come and go within a few hours.

Who hasn't had either poison ivy or poison oak or known someone who has had it badly enough to be miserable? The terrible rash and even open sores that can come from exposure to either plant can lay you low for weeks and, in severe cases, for months. How many times has a housewife had a persistent rash, only to learn it came from a beautiful house plant someone gave her as a gift or gesture of friendship. A rash from a house plant is difficult to detect because you may only come in direct contact with the plant once or twice a week when watering it. Consequently, it may take months before the source of the rash is detected.

Other people have had persistent skin rashes, only to learn, after going from doctor to doctor, that it was a kidney disorder or a complicated spleen problem that brought it on. In writing the book *Eating Right For A Bad Gut*, I interviewed a hundred people with Crohn's disease or various types of inflammatory bowel disease, and learned that most intestinal flare-ups are preceded for several days or a week by a mild skin rash. These rashes most often start on the legs, but also begin on the scalp, chest, back, and sometimes in the mouth as mild canker sores.

Some special functions of the skin include protecting your organs from the environment, and regulating body temperature and body water content. The skin is elaborately endowed with a nerve system that senses changes in the environment. To fulfill its roles, the skin has an intricate blood supply, a nervous system that is particularly sensitive, and a system of sweat glands that can release or retain water, as necessary, to keep the body temperature constant. Some nerves in the skin are attached to hairs, so they combine to form a lever system that is extremely sensitive to touch. If you become scared, these hairs will stand straight up and become about ten times as sensitive. You can see how responsive this system is by simply touching a few hairs on your arm.

You can prove how porous your skin is by having someone rub the oil of a crushed garlic clove on the bottom of your foot. You'll soon have a garlic taste in your mouth. If someone eats a lot of garlic or onions, their skin will smell. Similarly, if they smoke regularly, eat lots of carrots or take beta carotene, their skin will change color. This proves you are what you eat or smoke, and your skin discloses what's going on inside your body.

My brief discussion only hints at what this marvelous organ does for us. But it also means that when the skin begins to act up, it can be the result of many things. Skin disorders such as Joshua's experience, can be from something we're eating or touching, a serious disease in some other part of our body, fumes we don't even notice, or even a metabolic disorder. The skin is simply giving an early warning signal of something more serious.

When a child gets a skin disorder it can be exceptionally complicated, because the child can't communicate as effectively with doctors. Consequently, everyone second guesses what's wrong or how the child feels. Joshua's story brings out the extreme frustration connected with a serious skin disorder. In this case, it turned out to be a metabolic problem that nutrition solved.

Most books, many doctors, and people will tell you that a rash is caused by "toxins in the blood." After all, it looks like a severe case of poison ivy or poison oak, which is directly related to toxic substances that get into the blood. But when a rash persists, the doctor knows it's the result of chemicals produced somewhere in the body that is causing the skin to react. The skin produces pustules, oozes a slime, and a rash develops. All are attempts by the skin to get rid of something toxic.

BACK TO JOSHUA

Pam tried to detoxify Josh by giving him Herb-Lax. She even tried an Herb-Lax poultice on his skin. If anything, Joshua just got worse. This was a clue to her, that whatever was causing the problem wasn't easily eliminated; or that his body was producing something so rapidly, that it was being replaced as fast as it was being eliminated.

It's an understatement to describe Joshua's irritating sensation as "itching." He would scratch and dig all night long. Both parents would take turns watching over him to keep the damage he inflicted on himself to a minimum. Even tying his hands wouldn't stop the process. Let Pam's words give you an idea of how persistent Joshua was to relieve the terrible pain. "If I held his hands so he couldn't scratch, he'd rub his elbows against his sides. His favorite was to rub his knees together because they seemed to be especially bad. His itching and irritation was worse around his joints. It took all my strength one night to pull his legs apart so he couldn't hurt himself." Can you imagine a person, over twice Joshua's size, using all her strength to pull his legs apart?

In retrospect, Pam realizes that most things they tried were like throwing gasoline on a fire. One doctor explained to them that the worst thing you can do for eczema is use "over-the-counter" products that say they are for eczema. When he told her this, she recalled that they had tried all of them and Joshua just got worse. Pam learned that any drug ending in "ane," just made Joshua worse, even though they claimed to relieve eczema.

As parents, we can only guess at the guilt this must have caused for Pam. We all want to do our best for our children and when they're ill, we become very anxious. Indeed, most parents would gladly change places with their sick child, because their love is so deep. So when you learn you've done the wrong thing, you're devastated.

Pam met adults who had similar problems or whose children had eczema. They all gave the same advice: "Stay away from doctors. They just make it worse." Most of them also said it was a nutrition problem. But Pam was using Shaklee products and so was Josh. If it was a simple nutrition problem with vitamins or protein, you couldn't prove it by Josh. No one would ever guess that Joshua's problem was a normal reaction because of something his body couldn't make. In short, it wasn't a toxic chemical being produced. It was a material *not* being produced. However, Pam's nutritional program probably saved Joshua's life, even if it didn't clear his symptoms.

In defense of the doctors, they had to deal with Joshua's symptoms. As you'll see later, we know now how the problem can be relieved, but in 1984 no one had any idea of an alternate nutritional approach. So it wasn't surprising that people said "stay away from doctors." They reacted this way because the medication appeared to do nothing and the stress of the doctor's office or clinic seemed to make it worse. Good intentions don't count when a child is sick.

Pam went to a chiropractor whose theory taught that Joshua's condition was the result of poor spinal-fluid circulation. The chiropractor tried various manipulations and natural remedies that helped, but produced no cigar. Joshua would appear to be a little better, and then get worse with a vengeance. The improvement from these attempts by the chiropractor probably falls into the category of "mind over matter."

Joshua's skin would ooze so badly that he'd always feel slimy. Since the attacks would come on at night, the bedclothes would be wet with a slime by morning. The sheets and pillowcases required daily washing. As you recall, both parents took turns trying to get Joshua to sleep and prevent him from scratching.

At this point I feel obliged to point out a clue that everyone missed. Pam repeatedly pointed out that the itching would start at night. An internist who is familiar with inflammatory diseases would have immediately realized that Josh was suffering from an inflammatory illness caused by some unknown factor. A careful family history should have revealed that Kerry had exhibited the same symptoms previously.

Joshua's skin was continually flaking and sloughing and became red like he had a bad sunburn. The dead skin would regularly come off in sheets, so Pam would vacuum the living room rug daily to remove the flaked skin. It was amazing how Joshua's recuperative powers were so undaunted; his little body kept going. This certainly was the result of good nutrition.

In hindsight, this incredible skin growth was a second clue to the inflammatory nature of Joshua's problem. However, it was also testimony to Pam's nutrition program for Joshua, which included protein and the generous use of Shaklee supplements. Without this nutrition, his body could never have mounted its reserves to keep fighting. For example, the skin normally reproduces itself every four weeks. In hindsight, Joshua's problem, later correctly diagnosed, indicates his skin was reproducing every four days; a confirmation of his nutrition and the body's restorative powers.

Joshua had a ravenous appetite. Most parents worry about their children eating. Not Pam. Josh couldn't get enough. He would eat several helpings of good food all day long. No wonder his skin could slough off and be replaced at a prodigious rate. Pam's nutrition kept his appetite going and his body working.

During this time Pam marveled at how quickly Joshua's body responded to his condition. He would wake up in the morning raw and red. Skin would flake off all day long, but his body kept fighting. The ooze continued to be produced in large quantities. His body was fighting a fierce battle, but no one could see the enemy.

Although she realized the doctors couldn't do anything, in desperation, she returned to Doctor Moore, the only one who had helped Joshua. The doctor examined Josh again and put his diagnosis in one short sentence: "He's the worst case I've ever seen in my entire career." She asked the doctor to hospitalize him to see if they could stabilize his condition. The answer was a short and sweet, "No. We can't do anything for him in a hospital and he would run the risk of getting a serious infection."

The doctor explained how the family, including

Joshua, would have to learn to live with the problem. At about this time, the word psoriasis came up. The doctor saw the clues and was starting to call the condition psoriasis. Joshua would have this for the rest of his life. He did observe that topical cortisone helped and that was about all they could do.

The fact that topical cortisone helped was proof that the skin was producing the ooze. The skin's response to the ointment probably confirmed to the doctor, a dermatologist, that what he observed was inflammation and irritation. But at the time, no one seemed to ask, "What's causing the inflammation?"

One of the things Pam tried giving Joshua was a natural diuretic, that the chiropractor thought would cleanse Josh's cells. The diuretic helped because it removed fluid. A professional massage was the only thing that actually gave Joshua a full night's sleep. Pam reasoned that Josh's little body was racked with stress and tension. Adults relax with a massage, so why not a four-year-old. She was so used to being up with him, that she simply sat up and watched him sleep all night after the massage. Again, this was an important clue; inflammation thrives on stress!

A turning point came by what, in retrospect, seems like God's way of helping people find each other. Pam was invited to speak at a Shaklee meeting in Florida. She decided to go. Her husband had a look of abject fear on his face when she announced her decision. Three days alone with Joshua was tough duty for anyone, even a parent who loved the little guy. It meant no sleep and constant work.

At the Florida meeting, Pam heard someone talk about how EPA helped relieve a skin problem. She got to thinking: "I'll give it a try. It surely can't hurt." Now, you've got to realize that this little boy was taking Instant Protein,

Vita-Lea, calcium-magnesium, Vita-C, and other supplements. So, although Pam was tuned into nutrition and believed in it, one more supplement was worth trying, but her skepticism was normal.

She actually had EPA on the shelf at home, but somehow she had associated it with blood cholesterol. Pam had reasoned that the last thing Joshua had to worry about was his cholesterol level. Therefore, she sold EPA to some of her customers, but didn't give any to Joshua.

She gave Joshua three EPA capsules immediately after returning from Florida. This kid was so desperate to help himself, that he chewed the EPA (that was before the fishy taste had been eliminated). Joshua had nerve! Within about one hour, he looked better. Pam gave him two more capsules. The red nodules he had in some places started to disappear. They actually watched them go away. In about a week, they settled on five EPA daily.

Within ten days, Joshua's eczema had cleared up so that he started looking normal. He could begin leading a regular life again. You've got to realize that, by this time, the eczema was so bad, that he couldn't walk properly. Consequently, Joshua had to start some things all over again at the age of four. He returned to little boyhood once more and started over.

After three months on EPA, Joshua's skin was completely cleared. Pam also heard that another essential oil, gamma linolenic acid (GLA), usually obtained in Evening Primrose Oil, also helped. She started Joshua on GLA as well. He showed even more improvement, so she kept him taking EPA and Evening Primrose Oil.

Final confirmation of his improvement came when she took Joshua back to Doctor Moore, the physician who helped Joshua the most and who also said he would have the problem for life. Doctor Moore said that his skin looked normal and that the psoriasis would always be there, but that it had gone into remission as a result of Pam's effort.

Joshua still has the psoriasis and will always have it, but it's dormant. Sometimes it flares up, and when it does, Pam gives him extra EPA and more GLA. This stops the flare-up and his life returns to normal.

WHAT'S GOING ON HERE?

In 1984 when all this started and EPA was introduced, we didn't know how important EPA could be. However, all hindsight is perfect vision and now I can explain what was going on.

Joshua was probably born with the tendency to have psoriasis, an inflammatory disease, that is a form of arthritis. His older sister Kerry had a similar, mild attack that was also diagnosed as eczema, but prompt steroid treatment stopped her attack and she returned to normal. There's a good chance her eczema was returning to normal by itself. With Joshua, circumstances were much worse.

Stress is a trigger for any inflammatory disease. In Joshua's case, the immunizations, living for a week away from home, and the idea of going to an unknown preschool was a triple whammy of stress for this four-year-old. These events got the psoriasis off to a running start. Add scratching, digging, and pain to the stress, and the disease accelerated. This acceleration is often characteristic of inflammatory illnesses. The things people do to relieve the pain often make the illness worse. I think of it as a downward spiral in which everything we do makes it worse.

Steroid injections, such as cortisone, will stop inflammation in adults. However, who's going to give a child with eczema cortisone shots? The side effects of the cure could be worse than the disease. After all, it's the skin we're dealing with and the rash could be the result of something he ate, an allergy, or myriad things. But the fact that topical cortisone creams worked, to some extent, is a clue.

The fact that the chiropractor's diuretic worked indicates that Joshua's body was full of things that kept the irritation going. Also, Joshua's response to the massage, which gave him a restful night, proves how big a role stress and anxiety play in aggravating the inflammation.

Enter EPA and GLA. Are these oils magic? Do they work miracles? Yes, they work miracles in some people, because they restore metabolism to normal. Both oils are converted in the body to prostaglandins that modulate inflammation. Indeed, in 1992, eight years later, both of these oils have been clinically tested in this conversion capacity and proven to be effective.

Our body produces three prostaglandins. One, PGE_2, antagonizes or increases inflammation as a defensive mechanism, and two others, PGE_1 and PGE_3, modulate inflammation. PGE_1 is produced from gamma linolenic acid (GLA) and in clinical studies has been proven to modulate inflammation, which is generated internally from what could be loosely called "toxins."

PGE_3 is produced from EPA and modulates inflammation by balancing PGE_2. In addition, EPA or its metabolic by-products have been clinically tested and shown to be effective in reducing both the severity of psoriasis, as well as other inflammatory illnesses, including arthritis and Crohn's disease, which is an inflammatory disease of the intestinal tract.

PGE_1, which antagonizes inflammation, is produced from most fat, especially meat and dairy products. Joshua's mother didn't feed him those foods, so you could ask why he was helped by EPA and GLA.

Although there's much active research in these fields, we know that some people don't make enough GLA, if they make any, but they respond to it very well when it's used as a supplement. In fact, a few diseases are completely cleared by GLA supplements. Clinical studies have proven it helps some people who have arthritis, so it follows that it should help some people who have psoriasis.

Although Joshua had an excellent diet, it didn't contain much EPA. By giving him EPA supplements, his mother pushed his metabolism to make the prostaglandin PGE_3 and other materials from EPA, the leukotrienes. Together they balance PGE_2 and modulate inflammation. Obviously, Joshua's body simply requires more of these materials than average to "push" his metabolism to make the correct prostaglandins. You could say, "It's in his genes."

IS HE CURED?

Joshua will always have psoriasis, even if it's dormant. His experience with EPA and GLA proves that the nutritional needs of people with these disorders are greater than those for average people. Will the EPA and GLA help the psoriasis remain dormant? Only time will tell. I'm betting it will.

Evening Primrose Oil is a substance that was discovered by the American Indians. Pilgrims of the Plymouth colony sent it back to England where it became known as the "king's cure-all." Indeed, it was one of the few direct economic-benefits to flow from the Plymouth colony to England. It was used for various therapeutic purposes up into the beginning of the 20th century when it was displaced by more sophisticated drugs. GLA is now entering into a renaissance as scientists begin using nutrition more seriously.

GLA is found in mother's milk. This proves it has an important role in infant health and nutrition. However, its only dietary sources are the seeds of obscure fruits, such as black currants, and other seeds of the "borage" plants. Active research on GLA suggests to me that it is an important "conditional" nutrient for many people.

CHAPTER

11 Fatigue and Malaise

LYKE'S STORY

Lyke won't hesitate when you ask her what day she remembers most clearly: "August 15, 1945." The day was remarkable because she had just turned nine and an American Thunderbolt fighter plane (P-47) flew over the "camp of living death" she was in. Lyke was in a Japanese concentration camp on her home island of Java, a Dutch possession before World War II. "We could see the pilot, he flew so low. Wind from the propeller blew up dust, shook the buildings, and the palm trees blew. The noise of the engine was so loud I thought my eardrums would burst. I was so inspired by this flight that I can tell you exactly where I stood, what I wore, who was with me, and what they wore. To the survivors in the camp, it meant deliverance. We knew the allies were winning the war and we would soon be delivered from the hell that we faced 24-hours every day."

When the Japanese took Java, Lyke's father had been forced to keep his coffee and quinine plantation going for the Japanese war effort. However, 20 months after they invaded, the Japanese decided all Dutch citizens should be placed in concentration camps. Lyke, her mother, and brother were sent to a camp for women and children, and her father was sent to a camp for men. Then, shortly after, her brother was separated into a labor camp for men over the age of 10. Yes, at that time and in that part of the world, boys 10-years-old were classified as men. The family wasn't reunited until 1946.

Life in the camps went from difficult, but survivable, to a grim, 24-hour-daily struggle to stay alive. People lost weight, became skinny, and finally looked like walking skeletons. Life was so delicate that any extra work, a simple illness, or a beating for any minor infraction could mean death. Lyke's mother got beriberi (a simple B-vitamin deficiency). By sharing their rations, Lyke and the other women kept her alive and out of the hospital. The camp hospital was not a place to restore health, but a place where they let you die. After the war, statistics showed that about 50 percent of Japanese prisoners died in the camps. This compares to about 1 percent in comparable German prisoner-of-war camps. Don't confuse these prisoner-of-war camps with the German death camps which were the basis of the holocaust.

Any source of protein in the camp disappeared — snails, rats, cats, dogs, large bugs, worms, and just about anything that crawled. Any animal kingdom member hapless enough to enter the camp became food. However, even that extra food wasn't nearly enough. Life hung by a thread, with death waiting as a friend in the shadows.

Dysentery caused by tropical parasites that thrived in the poor water and on the unwashed food given to the prisoners, was a constant reality with people living in the camp. Add the use of excrement for fertilizer, and conditions were right for chronic illness and epidemics. Diarrhea that accompanies the dysentery, brings the secondary problem of dehydration. Dehydration increases fatigue and makes a person more susceptible to the ravages of malnutrition. Fatigue had the other possibility of making you look lazy and become a candidate for a beating. A beating was usually a prelude to death.

Lyke often felt weak. Starch, once used to press shirts, became food. Now she realizes that her constant fatigue was from not enough nutrients, including protein. Lyke also remembers pounding headaches that today she knows were consistent signs of B-vitamin deficiency. Ironically, the people in the camp divided a rare Red Cross food-package containing a meal for one person among about 25 people. Even her small share was too much food for Lyke to tolerate at one time in her weakened condition. She had become so skinny and her stomach so small that food had to be parcelled out in small doses. Food was divided among the people with a small, delicate Dutch teaspoon, which is one-third the size of an American teaspoon.

Shortly after Jan Banning, the Dutch pilot flying for the U.S. Air Force, had buzzed Camp Lampersari on August 15th, 1946, the island was liberated. At first, Lyke, her mother, and brother were placed in what had been a Japanese army camp where they were, at last, given enough food. From there they were transported across the island and reunited with her father. Somehow, the entire family had survived. In contrast to their good fortune, two of her uncles, who were placed in the same camp with her father, died. Two out of three survivors were typical for men in the camps.

Lyke's mother was in such bad condition, in spite of being given enough food, that Amercian and Dutch army doctors decided to send the family back to Holland for better medical facilities. Lyke remembers the stopover in Egypt, because they were given blankets for use in Holland where it was cold. Lyke still has her blanket as a reminder of kindness in another time. When they reached Holland, Lyke was the first person at the door of the plane to see the waving crowds. She said, "Mommie, mommie, there is a fat man waiting for us." The "fat man" was her slender uncle. In contrast to the slender uncle who had also survived the German occupation, Lyke and her family were skin and bones.

In spite of double rations and efforts by the Dutch doctors, Lyke's mother died in 1948 at the age of 42. Her body had simply been deprived past the point of no return. No matter how much food she ate, and how hard the doctors tried, her body couldn't rebuild itself. She simply couldn't extract enough nourishment from food.

One could ask, "Why did she survive the camp only to perish in the midsts of adequate food and medical care?" Of course we'll never know, but we can speculate that it has to do with the human spirit and a mother's determination to save her family. When that job was complete, it seems her body said, "It's okay to go now." Other families didn't fare so well. Lyke's family had an inner source of stamina that kept them all going, because the odds predicted that only two of them would make it back. As it was, four made it until 1948.

Lyke and her brother lived with several families in Holland for a time. She even lived in a girl's school in Holland. Indonesian prisoner-of-war children without mothers were often shifted from family to family. Lyke's dad and other men returned to Indonesia to start rebuilding what was once a thriving economy. This complex family relationship imposed a great deal of stress on a teenage girl who was still recovering from serious malnutrition and the loss of her mother. Now that her father was half a world away, she had to accept the fact that she was a guest wherever she stayed. Lyke learned to get along and not complain.

You have to realize that Holland itself was recovering from devastation and starvation, but the Dutch government did everything it could for its citizens. Help came from the Marshall Plan and other war relief efforts. Exprisoner-of-war children, like Lyke, were given double rations to help them return to normal.

In spite of having plenty to eat, Lyke never really felt good. She had no energy, was always tired, and longed for evenings to come so she wouldn't be criticized for sleeping. Her gums often bled when she ate crusty bread or hard crackers and during the night when she slept. Both were definite signs of poor health from prolonged deprivation.

At 18, Lyke and a girl friend toured England as a celebration. One day of sightseeing called for a day of rest. This tiredness concerned her friend so, on her advice, Lyke's dad requested she be given a complete physical.

"I can't find anything wrong," was the doctor's report. But Lyke knew the fatigue was real. She couldn't shake it even though she looked okay to the doctors. In fairness, the doctors of 1954 were dealing with many unknowns at the time. Never in history had so many people been so completely deprived for so long. A few vitamins and minerals were still being discovered. So when the doctors compared Lyke's health to other young women of the same age who had been living under poor conditions, she fell into that range they called "normal." Their criteria were based on weight, height, blood pressure, pulse rate, and other such measures. In 1992, doctors have more knowledge and look for other indicators.

By the age of 30, Lyke not only felt tired all the time, she looked tired all the time. The corners of her lips were always cracked, her complexion was poor, and she had frequent diarrhea. In spite of this, Lyke kept going—she called on the same reserves she needed to survive in the Japanese concentration camp. No matter how she felt, she moved forward. She lived in this state of health until the age of 38.

In November 1974, Lyke was introduced to Shaklee food supplements. After one week of taking Vita-Lea and Instant Protein, she noticed two things: she wasn't tired and the cracks around her mouth were almost gone. Lyke had found a solution to her problems. Within a month her complexion had color, she looked younger, healthier, and felt better than she could ever remember. No more faking energy. No more saying "yes" to an invitation when her mind said "no!" Her hair had body, her gums stopped bleeding, and she jumped out of bed in the morning. Life had the same joy she remembered it had in 1942 before the Japanese took over her island.

IS IT IN LYKE'S HEAD?

No! We know today that Lyke and countless others left prison camps with an intestinal problem that will never clear. We call this problem malabsorption—literally sick absorption. These people can absorb the fat and calories from food, but not enough of the vitamins and minerals that make everything work. In short, they're getting food, but not nutrition.

A few clues are pertinent: bleeding gums are usually a sign of inadequate vitamin C and some B vitamins; cracks at the corners of the mouth are sure signs of B-vitamin deficiency; both C-vitamin and B-vitamin deficiencies cause fatigue. In addition to lack of vitamins C and B, a shortfall in iron and zinc completed the picture.

Malabsorption probably accounts for these nutrient shortfalls. In the concentration camp Lyke had developed dysentery, which damaged the absorptive capacity of her small intestine. In the camp it was normal to be constantly fatigued and have symptoms of deficiency. For some inmates, once they returned to freedom, simply getting enough food solved the problem. Other inmates never recovered, no matter how much food they ate. Lyke's mother is a good example of that. Chance led Lyke to the only solution for malabsorption: supplementation.

Vita-Lea, a complete supplement, overcame Lyke's nutrient need by mass action. Mass action is a simple process that is built on the idea that if you absorb a small percentage of a nutrient, simply getting more will solve the problem, because a small percentage of a lot is enough.

Instant Protein gave Lyke's body two things. First, she got enough high quality protein as essential amino acids to restore and rebuild tissues. Simultaneously, Instant Protein provides an excess of nonessential amino acids that her body could use as energy. In addition, it gave a dose of more B vitamins necessary to keep her metabolic machinery running. Not surprising, by simply taking both Vita-Lea and Instant Protein, Lyke got a new lease on life.

When I interviewed Lyke, I got another impression that I can't quantify. Along with the supplements came an optimistic spirit. She had been raised in a spirit of optimism that was broken by the war and then obliterated by her mother's death. At Shaklee meetings an optimism came into her life with the supplements. An optimistic outlook with unquestionable nutrition is an unbeatable combination.

Today, almost 50 years after her ordeal began, Lyke is a mature, energetic woman, who shares her good fortune with others. She uses many supplements, is tireless, and never feels fatigued. Her eyes sparkle, complexion glows, and she radiates sunshine wherever she goes.

CHAPTER

12 High Blood Pressure

CARLA'S STORY

"I had some occasional dizzy spells and a nosebleed now and then, but I tried not to let them interfere with anything. Friends said they were probably caused by a food allergy, air pollution, or perhaps a hormonal imbalance. They didn't want to say I was overweight. I went to give blood for a friend whose son was going into surgery, and was told by the nurse that I couldn't give blood because my blood pressure was 150 over 110! She advised me to see a doctor right away." At the time, Carla was a 36-year-old mother of two girls and was overweight.

The next day Carla took the blood-bank nurse's advice and went to see her doctor whom she had not seen in about five years. Carla's doctor, a woman, confirmed that her blood pressure was, in fact, high and advised prompt treatment with medication. She gave Carla a routine physical that included being weighed, having blood and urine samples taken, as well as the usual poking and probing. The doctor didn't see any complications and concluded it was high blood pressure—hypertension (the medical term). Carla's experience with high blood pressure is typical.

Carla continued her story. "The doctor put me on medication because my pressure was so high, but she recommended I try diet. She said my blood pressure would probably drop to normal if I would lose about 25 pounds. I'm five feet four inches and weighed 160 pounds at the time; I was fat. The doctor also felt I'd have to follow a low-salt diet as well as a reducing diet. So, I left the office with a printed diet and a brochure that explained how to cut out dietary salt."

Carla soon learned that medication for high blood pressure had a double cost connected to it. You paid the druggist over a dollar a day and you also paid by feeling strange. At first she felt nauseous, but most medicine gave her a queasy feeling. Sometimes she would get a lightheaded feeling, but a couple of times she blacked out briefly when she stood up from sitting. Her doctor had warned her of this and adjusted her medication until the dose level kept the side effects to a minimum, but still kept her blood pressure within the normal range. The doctor kept reminding Carla about losing weight and following a low-salt program. However, once the medication was right, there was no need to speak with the doctor, so his diet prompting stopped.

"I never used a salt shaker again, but the brochures weren't clear on the amounts of salt in other foods. It didn't say 'don't eat this or that.' The booklet talked of sodium in some foods and salt in other foods, but seemed to skirt the issue. I followed the diet for a week and lost a couple of pounds, but I didn't have the time or the drive to prepare three sets of meals for my family: one for me, one for the girls, and one for my husband Tony. Consequently, I tried to eat what they ate, but I just ate less. Face it, the diet wasn't working. The drugs worked and I got used to the side effects, but I never felt right using the drugs. I know it isn't clear when I say I didn't feel right, but that's the way I felt. I think it was psychological."

HIGH BLOOD PRESSURE

High blood pressure is called the "silent killer" because it has no firm symptoms. The vague symptoms Carla felt are about all that anyone ever notices. And who doesn't have a headache now and then? High blood pressure probably causes more deaths indirectly than any other illness outside of overweight. High blood pressure dramatically increases the likelihood of stroke, heart attack, kidney failure, blindness, and a number of other less deadly, but serious health problems.

About one in five American and Canadian adults have high blood pressure. By age 65, about three in five adults have high blood pressure; some studies argue it's three in four. About 50 percent of these people know they've got the illness and are being treated by a physician with medication. The other 50 percent don't realize they are ill. Remember, it's usually a symptomless disease. If you don't get a physical, you often don't know you have hypertension. That's why it's a silent killer.

About 80 percent of all high blood pressure can be completely controlled by diet. The other 20 percent of people who have high blood pressure can reduce their medication if they also follow the correct diet. In order, the dietary requirements to reduce blood pressure are weight, alcohol, salt reduction, sodium-potassium balance, calcium adequacy, and EPA. People with real difficult cases of high blood pressure need to follow a very low-sodium diet of less than 300 to 500 milligrams of sodium daily. Any expert, including the surgeon general, says diet should be the first line of attack and is, by far, the treatment of choice.

High blood pressure has a hereditary tendency. You inherit the tendency to get it and the environment brings it on. Food, alcohol, and stress are all part of the environment that causes blood pressure to go up. Because of heredity, about 15 percent of people with high blood pressure won't ever succeed with diet and will always require medication. These people are easily identified by a physician who specializes in this illness.

Stress is a large factor in causing blood pressure to rise. In fact, people in some occupations and those with certain personality types are more likely to have high blood pressure. But even these people can use techniques, which include exercise, meditation, biofeedback, and others, to control their problem. It seems that only about 15 percent of all hypertensives absolutely require medication. Why then, don't more people use diet to control high blood pressure? Carla put it nicely when she said, "It's tough to take off weight." Following a low-salt diet or balancing sodium and potassium correctly isn't easy and calls for a serious commitment.

In my book *The High Blood Pressure Relief Diet*, I have explained low sodium and sodium-potassium balance, and have provided dietary plans, recipes, and advice. It's an easy book to use and was chosen as one of the best diet books of 1989. Anyone with high blood pressure owes it to themselves to, at the the very least, try dietary control. All it calls for is some self discipline, will power, and a desire to be healthy.

BACK TO CARLA

"A friend told me about a dietary plan that someone she knew had followed and lost 20 pounds. Besides, her friend now sells the products," Carla said and quickly added, "and I was desperate. I had tried all the fad diets but gave into my 'making three meals for each meal' problem. When Helen's friend called, I was willing to see her."

Carla was introduced to Shaklee products. When the distributor learned Carla had high blood pressure, she told her about a nutrition seminar she had attended, where a home-office expert, using slides, showed how well the diet program worked for high blood pressure—people lost weight and high blood pressure at the same time. The distributor introduced Carla to the basic supplements and especially EPA and calcium, because this expert had said they helped reduce high blood pressure. Carla was now equipped with everything she needed.

"I wrote out a check for almost $150. It was the best investment of my life. I ate two meals a day of Shaklee Slim Plan and a large salad for the third meal. I also took the supplements, including fiber and Herb-Lax. I ate dinner with the family; it's just that they had a 'rabbit' at the table." Carla laughed when she reflected on the process.

"Although I lost only 11 pounds in the first two weeks, I felt like I had dropped all 25 pounds. Things weren't tight on me anymore. In the third week of my Shaklee diet I felt so good, that I went off the medication for two days and had my blood pressure taken at the drug store where they have a machine. I know these machines aren't so accurate, but my blood pressure kept reading 135 over 85. I spent $1.25 for each reading and it was always just about the same." Carla even sounded excited talking about it later.

When Carla went back to her doctor to have her blood pressure measured, the doctor congratulated her and said she had succeeded in controlling her high blood pressure by diet. She also warned her that if she didn't keep the weight off and her salt intake down, the high blood pressure would return.

It's about four years since Carla started using the Shaklee Slim Plan and supplements. Now her entire family uses Shaklee products and she even distributes them. Carla has not had any problem with high blood pressure nor has she had difficulty with her weight. She lost the entire 25 pounds and then another 10 pounds. Today she weighs a healthy 125 pounds.

RAY'S STORY

"I wasn't overweight! I had to work to get my blood pressure down." Ray describes his problem very dramatically. His delivery commands your attention.

"I followed a supplement plan that included Vita-Lea, EPA, and gobs of all the other supplements. I had heard that EPA, calcium and magnesium are important, so they were my standbys." Ray had also purchased a copy of my book *The High Blood Pressure Relief Diet* and followed a low-sodium, high-potassium diet. In his words: "I earned my low blood pressure the hard way! And I keep it low the same hard way!" Modesty is not Ray's problem. His blood pressure runs about 125 over 75 to 80, which, his doctor agrees, is excellent.

Ray continued, "At 40, I had been told I would be on high blood pressure medication for life. I hated it and owe my success to Shaklee products and my dietary program." Today Ray is the picture of health and you'd never know he has a blood pressure problem. He jogs several miles at a time regularly and is also an enthusiastic tennis player.

WHAT'S GOING ON HERE?

These two people represent the extremes of dietary and dietary-supplement control of high blood pressure. Each one of them is at one end of what I call the "dietary spectrum."

Carla was probably hypertensive because of her weight. With excess weight, the body becomes insulin in-sensitive. Not all overweight people have this problem. For reasons not well understood, the kidneys respond by elevating blood pressure through a complex mechanism that involves salt reabsorption, as well as the production of a hormone-like substance. The bottom line of these two actions is that people like Carla respond quickly to weight loss and moderate salt reduction. Their blood pressure drops as soon as they bring their weight into line.

Shaklee Slim Plan drink mix is a moderate salt product. So, if people follow the plan and don't add salt to their food, they are on a salt-restricted diet, that also provides more than enough potassium. With weight loss, this mineral balance in the Slim Plan brings blood pressure down quickly for people like Carla. Consequently, Carla saw results which seemed almost too good to be true. In reality, they're typical.

In addition to the weight loss and the mineral balance in the diet drink, Carla gained some benefit from the supplements. In this case, the critical supplements are EPA and calcium-magnesium. Vita-Lea also provides calcium and magnesium, but the body actually needs more than Vita-Lea provides, so the separate calcium-magnesium supplement is necessary.

EPA has been clinically tested in a number of studies in several countries and helps reduce blood pressure in two ways: it reduces the friction of the blood cells and the tension within the blood vessels; it also reduces intra-blood-vessel inflammation. EPA doesn't have a major effect on blood pressure, but it contributes to its reduction. Every millimeter of blood pressure reduction helps.

Inadequate dietary calcium seems to moderately elevate blood pressure in some people. When these people use calcium supplements, their blood pressure usually returns to normal. Magnesium seems to work in concert with calcium and has a modest effect on blood pressure. Some people speak of some magic ratio of calcium to magnesium. Hogwash to some ratio! If you get at least the RDA of calcium and magnesium, you will not have high blood pressure that's traceable to either mineral.

Ray, in contrast to Carla, needed to reduce his sodium intake to less than 800 milligrams daily and keep his salt intake to a minimum. Sodium is part of salt, but so is the other side, chloride. Sodium, in the absence of chloride, can be tolerated much better by the body than sodium chloride, or salt. That's why some foods, such as milk, contain sodium, but are okay in moderation because they don't contain chloride. But the same level of sodium, as salt, would be a "no-no" on a low-sodium diet.

Ray benefited from the EPA for the reasons I mentioned and similarly benefited from calcium and magnesium. He could also use Shaklee Slim Plan drink mix as a meal substitute, but his major strategy required the plan I carefully developed in *The High Blood Pressure Relief Diet*. There really wasn't any substitute in his case, and Ray did, indeed, earn his results.

Most people who have high blood pressure are not as clearly separated as Ray and Carla. Average folks are moderately overweight with sodium and chloride sensitivity. They will still succeed in lowering their blood pressure if they do what Carla did. Black people are especially sensitive to chloride. This genetic disadvantage leaves them no choice but to follow the dietary program in detail.

CHAPTER

13 Hypoglycemia (Low Blood Sugar)/Diabetes

EARL'S STORY

"I would become irritable every morning at about ten o'clock and have a cup of coffee with a sweet roll. In about 20 minutes I would feel good again and people in the office wouldn't avoid me. My cantankerous performance would repeat itself in the afternoon about 2:30 or 3:00 o'clock. Virginia, my secretary, solved it for me with a cup of coffee and a snack.

This pattern of life was the old good news and bad news story. The good news: By eating, I kept from biting people's heads off. The bad news: I got increasingly overweight.

One day at work had been particularly stressful. There was no time for my customary coffee break and roll. I vividly remember looking at my watch—it was 11:30 A.M.—I got up from my desk and passed out right there. I woke up with a rescue-squad fireman strapping me onto a stretcher on wheels.

In the hospital my doctor made it very clear: 'Earl,

you've got what we call hypoglycemia—that's low blood sugar.' He then went on to explain how I produced too much insulin, which caused my blood sugar to drop. His solution: 'Carry a package of hard candy and keep sucking on one. It will keep your blood sugar up.'

He was right. My disposition changed—no more anxious periods or irritable actions with employees, but I got a little heavier. By now my five-foot eleven-inch frame was supporting about 230 pounds.

My doctor's solution was fine during the day, but by about 9:30 in the evening I was either asleep in front of the TV, or in bed building 'ZZZZZs.' I didn't realize what an effect this had on my wife. Our social life had dropped to zero.

One morning at breakfast, my wife Nancy told me that a friend had said I was treating my high blood sugar all wrong. Her friend had been to a Shaklee meeting where the topic was discussed, and she told Nancy that the worst thing for low blood sugar is sugar. This didn't make any sense to me, and I repeated what my doctor had said. She answered by putting a can of Instant Protein and a bottle of Vita-Lea on the table. She asked me if I would at least try the protein and Vita-Lea every morning for a week and not eat any candy or sweet rolls before noon. To keep peace in the family and preserve 15 years of marriage, I agreed, but I wouldn't let her mess with my cup of coffee, no how.

Following this plan wasn't any fun. I felt bloated, I burped, and wasn't hungry at lunch, but I got through the morning without candy and rolls, and just one cup of Virginia's excellent coffee. I decided it was a case of mind over matter and the effects would pass within a week.

By the end of the week I noticed two definite changes.

I had lots of energy all morning. In fact, I could go until about 2:30 p.m. without a snack. That's the good news. The bad news was that I felt constipated.

Nancy's friend had an answer for that, too. She said the extra nutrients I was getting caused mild constipation and she had just the solution: Herb-Lax. She told me to take one-or-two each day. She even showed Nancy how to brew an Herb-Lax tea with a little alfalfa thrown in. This was crazy! I told her alfalfa was for horses. She pointed out—correctly I might add—that I wasn't eating any more candy. I hadn't even noticed.

Nancy suggested another test: 'Why not have Virginia mix you an Instant Protein about noontime, just before lunch?' This was a conspiracy. I agreed because I was feeling quite good and noticed that my pants were just a tad looser. I decided to give it the 'old college try.'

Another week of twice-a-day Instant Protein and I felt great. Nancy and I went to a movie one night and I didn't fall asleep. I started watching Johnny Carson—he comes on at 11:30 P.M. I finally worked up the nerve to weigh myself. I was down to 220 pounds and I hadn't even been on a diet.

Nancy was overdoing it, however. She had me taking Vita-Lea, B-Complex, vitamin C, and drinking a tea made with Herb-Lax and alfalfa. I became concerned that my hair would turn green and I would either 'neigh' like a horse or 'moo' like a cow. Nancy said neighing was okay, but if I mooed, she'd cut back on the alfalfa."

WHAT'S GOING ON HERE?

Earl is typical of many people all over the world. They get caught in a vicious circle where they almost become their own worst enemy. Everyone giving him advice was right in some ways and wrong in others. Fortunately for Earl, his wife listened to the right person and he followed her advice.

Low blood sugar results from the body producing too much insulin. Insulin is a hormone that helps blood sugar, glucose, get inside the body cells where it's used for energy. When our blood sugar rises after a meal or a snack, the pancreas releases some insulin, so it will be metabolized for energy. The object is for just enough insulin release so the blood sugar will return to normal. Normal is from 80 to 110 milligrams of glucose per deciliter of blood. Each person has a level in this range, that's normal for them. However, in some people, and for some dietary reasons in all people, too much insulin is sometimes produced and their blood glucose will drop below 80. Normally the body responds by mobilizing a storage form of glucose called glycogen, that causes the blood glucose to bounce back to normal.

However, blood sugar doesn't always respond so well. Sometimes the blood sugar remains low and this sends a signal to the brain. Our brain relies almost exclusively on glucose for energy. Unlike other tissues, it doesn't use fat, and only some parts of the brain can use a few aminoacids for energy. So, when blood sugar drops below a level the brain considers normal, it becomes concerned.

The initial symptom of low blood sugar is anxiety. Anxiety causes most people to eat, and eating sets things right for the brain. However, if you're like Earl, you couldn't eat, because you have to set an example, or your job won't allow it until a normal coffee-break. So, the next action is for other centers in the brain to swing into action. Irritability is the next outward symptom. In short, the person is hard to get along with.

When blood sugar drops low enough, you can literally pass out, like Earl did. This is rare, however, because people usually eat when they get the early symptom of anxiety.

A common outcome of low blood sugar, hypoglycemia, is overweight. Overweight, like in Earl's case, develops because the person and the people around the person realize, that if you keep eating, the anxiety and irritability never develops. But this excess weight creates two long-term problems: diabetes and high blood sugar.

As weight increases, the body's cells become less sensitive to insulin. Consequently, the pancreas compensates by producing more insulin. Eventually, the pancreas can't keep up with the demand and medication is required. Initially the medication is used to prod, or boost the pancreas to produce more insulin. Finally, the pancreas becomes exhausted, and the person needs to take insulin by injection.

A secondary problem develops because, in some people, the kidneys respond to excess insulin by not performing their task correctly. When the kidneys go awry from insulin, high blood pressure results. Hence, the diabetes is complicated by a need for more medication to treat high blood pressure.

Several dietary solutions will bring this vicious hypoglycemic cycle into line. Get your weight down to normal! Don't eat foods that contain sugar without fiber!

Follow a high-protein diet! I'll review each of these solutions in detail.

Earl's doctor was correct when he said Earl needed sugar. He was wrong when he told him to eat candy or, in reality, sugar. He should have told him to eat an apple, a carrot, or some other fruit; protein would have been an even better recommendation. Fruits and vegetables contain simple sugars cloaked in a fiber matrix, that releases them into the blood slowly. Somehow the slow release of sugar is a signal to the pancreas to moderate its insulin production, so it doesn't overshoot its target.

Protein, especially Instant Protein, supplies amino acids. Some amino acids are used inside the cell for energy and don't require insulin. Hence, you get energy without using your circulating blood-glucose. This energy from Instant Protein is sustained over a long period and doesn't cause an insulin surge, or blood-sugar drop. Consequently, Earl found that he didn't need the candy or sweet roll and probably didn't even need the coffee.

Finally, people who are overweight and hypoglycemic owe it to themselves to lose weight. Excess weight taxes all the systems, but especially the pancreas and kidneys. Adult-onset diabetes — diabetes that develops in adults — is usually the result of the hypoglycemic's excess eating cycle. Maintaining normal weight is absolutely essential for these people to achieve good health.

RETURN TO EARL

Earl continued losing weight, but decided to go for it more aggressively, so he followed the Shaklee Slim Plan and brought his weight down to 185 pounds. He continues using Instant Protein, the supplements, and following a good diet.

His diet falls into the low-fat, high complex-carbohydrate category. A diet like this includes lots of vegetables, pasta, fruit, and other foods that are high in fiber and complex carbohydrates. He selects low-fat meats, such as chicken and fish, so he doesn't waste calories and risk putting weight on again.

Earl continues to work ten- to twelve-hours a day and has as much energy at the end of the day as he does at the beginning. He and Nancy spend more time together, go out regularly, and he never falls asleep in front of the TV or at the movies.

MARILYN'S STORY

Marilyn is a lovely lady, younger than Earl, who was trapped in the hypoglycemic cycle. Her doctor gave her a glucose-tolerance test and concluded she had all the symptoms of hypoglycemia. His approach was much better than Earl's doctor's, but flawed for another reason.

"He told me to eat lots of small meals of high-protein foods, like cheese," Marilyn said. So, she snacked on cheese, ate hamburgers without a roll, and, in general, shifted to a low-carbohydrate, high-protein, high-fat diet. She kept her blood sugar normal, but also kept her weight up as well. At about five-foot six-inches, Marilyn weighed over 180 pounds, but her blood sugar was normal. She exchanged hypoglycemia for looking like a blimp.

She finally took the same course that Earl did: Instant Protein, and the Slim Plan to get her weight down. She now weighs 130 pounds. Marilyn's task was much more difficult that Earl's, because she had to shift from high-fat foods, such as cheese, to high complex-carbohydrate vegetables, like potatoes, with sour cream, or broccoli. When you haven't eaten a lot of fruit and vegetables, it's tough to get started. Here's how Marilyn put it. "There were times when I craved hot-dogs with mustard like an ex-smoker craves a cigarette; or I wanted to sit down with a big chunk of cheddar cheese. Somehow, an apple just didn't have the mouth feel that I wanted. But after about a year, I found the foods that I used to crave, repulsive. In fact, if I eat a hamburger now, it feels all slippery and full of fat."

IS IT IN THEIR HEADS?

No. Earl and Marilyn are typical examples of many people. Food is all around us and most of it is the kind of food that contains sugar without fiber, or sugar with very little protein. Alternatively, it's mostly fat. Most food advertising is directed at foods with little or no nutritionally redeeming features, except low calories or low fat.

This trend is not confined to the United States. On a train ride on Japan's "bullet train" from Tokyo to Kyoto, a 3-hour drive, you are presented with food for sale, on average, every three to five minutes. A few of the offerings are fine; for example, fruit, but most of the items offered are high-sugar snacks.

Some people would say that artificial sweeteners are the answer. They aren't. All they do is provide the illusion of sweetness without the calories and have nothing to do with how we get our calories. We still require fiber, carbohydrates, protein, and some fat, all in the correct proportions. These requirements necessitate good food choices. Making things sweet doesn't fulfill the need, and may actually give young people, especially children, the wrong impression about food, if not life in general.

ADULT-ONSET DIABETES

Warren's Story

Warren had probably been hypoglycemic most of his life, even though it had never been diagnosed by a doctor. He compensated for the problem by snacking frequently in between meals. By the age of 45, he was overweight, with a somewhat large midsection—in other words, he had a big gut. The ratio of his waist to hip measurements would probably have been closer to two than one. You can figure out this ratio by measuring your hips and waist with a tape measure, and then dividing your waist measurement by your hip measurement. For good health, the ratio should be less than one.

When your waist to hip ratio is just over one, you've got a slight paunch; at a ratio of two, you're fat. The higher the ratio, the greater the paunch. A paunch is a good predictor of a person who is likely to get adult-onset diabetes as they approach 50 years and older. Adult-onset diabetes is often called Type II diabetes.

"I had a physical at work and the doctor said he didn't like my blood sugar level. The sugar showed up first in my urine, so he did a blood test. The doctor put me on a diet and followed up every two weeks for about six weeks. Same result: high," Warren said. He also admitted that he didn't do well with the diet. I asked him if he felt sick or had any symptoms.

"I was thirsty all the time. A drink of water only quenched the thirst for a few minutes. The doctor told me this was consistent with high blood sugar and adult-onset diabetes."

Warren tried to stick with the diet, but like many people, it's hard to follow a diet when there's no obvious reason. He couldn't stick with it well enough to get his weight down more than a few pounds, compared to the 30 pounds the doctor wanted him to lose. Consequently, the only solution was to take drugs. Oral medication, not insulin, kept Warren's blood sugar within acceptable limits. However, it took the threat of big-league medication to convince Warren that nutrition was worth a serious try. A conversation with his doctor, after being on oral medication for one year, was the jolt that got him started on nutrition.

"He didn't like the way my blood sugar kept creeping up and suggested I might have to go on insulin injections. I had gained back the few pounds I had lost plus a few more, and hadn't been watching my diet. Since I was taking drugs, I didn't think I'd have to worry and became complacent about what I ate. However, the thought of giving myself insulin was more than I could handle." Warren still sounds apprehensive when describing the idea of giving himself insulin injections.

Warren's wife took charge. She bought enough Shaklee Slim Plan to put him on a strict diet plan. His regimen included two Slim Plan drink mixes daily and one meal which was almost vegetarian. She also let him have fish and chicken. The weight started coming off. If he cheated, he would have Slim Plan three times a day. His wife didn't compromise on the program.

"I followed this plan for six months. I also took Vita-Lea, B-Complex, vitamin C and Daily Fiber Blend. I lost, on average, just over one and a half pounds each week. In the first few weeks the pounds went off fast, then the weight loss slowed down. In six months I was 36 pounds lighter. I was doing so well, that I decided to lose 15 more pounds. I felt better than I had in 20 years."

After losing about 25 pounds, Warren was able to stop medication. His blood sugar stayed in the normal range without the drugs. His doctor encouraged him to maintain his diet program even if he didn't lose any more weight.

Warren shifted from taking Slim Plan to taking Instant Protein as he became trim once again. Now his waist to hip ratio is just over one, which is fine for him, after all the years of being fat. He feels fine. He doesn't stress his body with excess weight or sugar. His daily plan consists of Instant Protein, Daily Fiber Blend, Vita-Lea, B-Complex, and other supplements. He has lots of energy, normal thirst patterns, and feels good.

"Now that I don't have high blood sugar, I can feel the old low blood sugar return if I don't eat right," he said. He was explaining that if he eats the wrong food, his body produces too much insulin and his blood sugar drops, anxiety returns, and his first thought is to eat something. His nutrition plan with Instant Protein and Daily Fiber Blend keeps this from happening.

DIABETES

Jean's Story

"I was told I was a diabetic at age 25. My doctor said I'm a 'brittle diabetic,' which I guess means it's tough to manage my blood sugar. He insisted I use insulin twice daily. I mixed two types of insulin because it seemed to work best. But I didn't like taking injections then, and I still don't."

As a young 33-year-old mother, Jean was aware of the fact that she'd be dependent on insulin all her life, but had lots of trouble keeping her blood sugar in line. She tried to follow a good diet and stick with diabetic exchange lists. But when she tried a Shaklee nutrition plan, she found out she could feel really good.

"I started on Instant Protein, took other supplements and Herb-Lax, and had more energy and felt better the first day. Pretty soon I was able to get along with about two-thirds my regular insulin."

Jean told her doctor everything she was doing. She expected trouble, because he always told her that she didn't need supplements. To her surprise, he encouraged her to keep the program going. He said she looked better than ever, he liked her spirit, and her tests were first rate. She promised him that she'd watch her blood sugar closely and experiment carefully.

"I found that if I used Instant Protein twice a day and ate vegetarian meals, I could get by with half my normal insulin. I regained the energy I had before I was declared a diabetic. Everyone noticed how good I felt and they remarked on how good I looked."

Jean learned something else about herself during her

experiments. She joined a health club. When she exercised regularly, used Instant Protein and Fiber Blend twice daily, she could get by on even less than half the insulin she had used before she started her nutrition plan. But that wasn't the best part. Sure, she had more energy, but she had no "highs" and "lows" that the doctor told her are characteristic of a "brittle" diabetic. Jean felt consistently good and had steady energy all day.

WHAT GOES ON HERE?

Warren and Jean are typical examples of two health-problem extremes, adult-onset diabetes and insulin-dependent diabetes, that are constantly increasing in our society. Since both of these problems are increasing faster than the population, and there is no germ causing them, something about our lifestyle is involved.

Many people who tend toward hypoglycemia when they're young, and gain weight like Warren did, become adult-onset diabetics when they're older. This happens because certain people become insulin insensitive when they gain weight. That means that their cells require more insulin than normal to use blood sugar effectively. A side effect of this problem is high blood pressure. Warren was typical, but the problem continues to strike people, especially men, a little younger each year.

Adult-onset diabetes comes in two forms. Either the pancreas doesn't produce enough insulin, or the body becomes insensitive to the insulin. If the person is slim, it's usually because the pancreas has run out of steam. If the person is overweight, the pancreas usually produces enough insulin, but the body's cells don't respond to its presence. Either case calls for more insulin output as a short-term solution. Diet is the long-term solution for overweight people. Slender people usually need medication.

Medication usually involves a drug which "kick starts" the pancreas into producing more insulin. This is fine for awhile, but after prolonged boosting, the pancreas runs out of steam. When the pancreas wears out, insulin injections are the only alternative left.

However, over 75 percent of adult-onset diabetes can be completely eliminated by getting the waist to hip ratio down to about one. In short, lose weight—return to a flat stomach and the correct weight. There's no compromise.

Protein is an ideal food program, because it provides much of its energy from the amino acids without a need for insulin. This means the body can get some energy without calling on the pancreas to produce more insulin.

Fiber is an ideal support supplement, because it modulates sugar as it enters the digestive tract. All food has some simple sugars, and fiber slows the rate at which these sugars enter the blood. This sends a signal to the brain that says "little sugar coming," and not the wrong signal, "big sugar load," so the body produces a modest amount of insulin at a slow rate. This helps prevent the low blood sugar that complicates the whole process.

Jean's case is typical of true diabetics that develop diabetes as adults. It's as if the pancreas just shuts down at a certain time. Sometimes the pancreas starts producing a little insulin from time to time. Jean's doctor did an excellent job of training her to manage her difficult case. By using two injections daily, she manages her blood sugar better and avoids many side effects of diabetes.

Once Jean started experimenting with nutrition, she

discovered that diet and insulin form an unbeatable team to manage diabetes. By using nutrition teamwork, her body has the energy it requires with minimum insulin. This reduces the side effects of diabetes even more. Teamwork involves protein, fiber, exercise, a good, high complex-carbohydrate diet, and a solid supplement plan.

It's teamwork because it keeps all body organs functioning at their optimal levels. And by keeping dietary fat to a minimum, Jean avoids the problems of high blood fat that usually dog diabetics as they get older. Two outcomes of the high-fat diet that many diabetics follow, is vision deterioration and cardiovascular disease, with a high risk of stroke.

CHAPTER

14 Lupus

CRYSTAL'S STORY

A young, healthy, active girl usually has her share of scratches and bruises. Crystal wasn't any different, but her scratches and bruises became infected more easily. Frequent bladder infections, a related problem, made her life difficult. As a young girl she had frequent visits to the doctor, and only once did he say to her mother, "Something is wrong with Crystal's blood. She gets too many infections." However, that was more of an observation than a diagnosis and they didn't follow up.

As a young mother, Crystal noticed that she'd get lumps of "knots" on various parts of her body, usually around her muscles. After a week or so they would disappear, so she just lived with them. At 23 years of age, a lump appeared on her abdomen and seemed to stay longer. "This seemed more serious, so I went to the doctor. He recommended a hysterectomy. Since I was 23 and wanted more children, I refused." The lump just disappeared after several months.

Crystal started having headaches and noticed that sometimes one of her joints would swell during the headache. One time the swelling would be in her fingers on one hand, and the next time it would be in a knee or an elbow. She sought the advice of an internist. "I asked him if there was a type of arthritis that could go from one joint to another and could be related to headaches?" At the time of her medical appointment, the swelling had gone down. It's like asking a talkative little child to show your friends how well they speak and all you get is silence!

After some questioning, the doctor decided her headaches were from birth-control pills. However, he concluded her joint swelling was not from birth-control pills, so he tested her for arthritis. This test, which looks for a protein called the "inflammation factor," requires a blood sample. The results of this finding are usually expressed as sedimentation rate, or "sed rate" for short. Crystal's arthritis test came back negative. The doctor said, "You don't have arthritis."

Now what should she do? She got headaches, knots or bumps in her muscles from time to time, and inflamed joints that seemed to come and go. By this time she, her friends, and family noticed that she always felt tired. She had been a person with lots of energy, but now she seemed to let her housework slide and took daily naps. Fatigue creeps up, so you don't really notice it. Crystal was taking a nap every morning and afternoon, but to make matters worse, she woke up tired even after a good night's sleep.

As the fatigue progressed, her eating habits became worse. She needed energy, so she ate candy. She was too tired to cook, so she ate food that came in boxes. Slowly, without realizing it, her diet shifted to sweets, packaged foods, and processed meat such as hot dogs. These eating habits didn't help whatever her health problem was.

Attacks became regular during a particularly traumatic period in her life. Her husband, a welder, had a work-related accident that required surgery and he couldn't work. Consequently, Crystal had to care for her three children and hold down a job in order to put food on the table. To add fuel to the fire, some friends who were in tough financial shape moved in with them to "get back on their feet"! Even though the friends did their share around the house, it was a tough, stressful way to live. Crystal was unable to get any quiet time.

Once her son was hurt in sports and required a trip to the doctor. When the doctor finished with her son, who was alright, she asked him to look at her inflamed hand. It hurt so much that she couldn't even hold a comb. The doctor thought it looked like active rheumatoid arthritis, so he took a blood test. It was negative! Crystal didn't have rheumatoid arthritis no matter how her hands looked and felt.

Before long, all her joints became swollen, and she couldn't hold eating utensils, open bottles, or comb her hair with her hands. It even hurt to walk. Something had to be done. Crystal and her husband packed into the car and went to a clinic that specialized in arthritis. By the time they arrived, most of the swelling had gone down and only her ankles were swollen. They were bad enough, so the clinic doctors took more blood tests. Once again, they were negative.

Even if the tests were negative, the doctors recognized the swelling and discomfort she was suffering, so they gave her prescriptions for a steroid, Butazolidin, a tranquilizer, Stelazine, and an antibiotic, Tetracycline. She decided not to take them. These prescriptions focused on what the doctors had concluded. They realized there was some inflammation, so they prescribed a steroid to make it stop. Since inflammation is stress related, they probably felt the tranquilizer would make things easier for her. Tetracycline knocks out a number of microorganisms, so the doctors probably thought she had a persistent low-grade infection, possibly in her digestive system, that caused the inflammation. Her decision not to take the drugs was wise.

Tetracycline can have serious side effects on a lupus patient. Since lupus hadn't been diagnosed, she could have died, because the doctors wouldn't have known what was happening. The Stelazine might have relaxed her, but it wouldn't have removed the stress, and Butazolidin isn't the correct steroid. If she lifted weights, she might have developed bigger muscles, but that's about all. The drugs alone would have increased her need for vitamins, but her diet had also become very poor by this time. Consequently, she was falling short nutritionally because of both her medication and diet.

Shortly after her visit to the clinic, the inflammation subsided, but something else took its place. One day she found it difficult to speak. Her next series of knots and bumps seemed to develop on her vocal cords. The doctors were at a similar loss to explain these symptoms and recommended speech therapy. They said the therapy would help her use what she had left. Speech therapy was like offering bottled water to someone whose house is on fire.

When rashes developed that would come and go on any part of her body, Crystal decided to consult with a new doctor in a larger city. She felt that doctors in large metropolitan areas treated more patients, so they would probably see things differently and be more apt to confer with each other.

Crystal went through another series of blood tests. This time the doctor had a hypotheses. He was looking for either rheumatoid arthritis or lupus and said jokingly: "Which would you rather have?" As if she had a choice and wasn't already frightened enough.

SYSTEMIC LUPUS ERYTHEMATOSUS

In 1960, lupus was one of those rare diseases that only a few specialists would talk about. Very few nonmedical people had ever heard of it. Now, in 1991, most people over the age of 55 have heard of lupus and many know someone who has it.

Lupus, more specifically, systemic lupus erythematosus, or SLE for short, means "the wolf." It's named the wolf because you can't predict what organ the disease will attack, and the flare-ups are savage.

BACK TO CRYSTAL

In the spring of 1981, Crystal was told that she had systemic lupus erythematosus (SLE). Right after being diagnosed, she got a serious kidney infection, along with a flare-up that totally immobilized her hand. Now that she knew what she had, she took the medication that the doctor prescribed and the flare-ups stopped.

It's important to realize that once a flare-up of lupus starts, it must be stopped. A runaway flare-up can be fatal. For example, consider Kay, who isn't with us any longer, even though she would be only 44 today. Her lupus flare-up got going, and by the time the doctors got started treating her, it was too late. Lupus is a big-league disease.

On a typical day, she might take four short naps and 24 aspirin, which caused ringing in her ears and stomach pain. Finally, when the pain became constant, she was put on Prednisone, an anti-inflammatory steroid. It stopped the inflammation, but the side effects were ferocious.

Crystal joined the Lupus Foundation, which sent her many booklets filled with lots of information about lupus. After reading them, she realized that all the symptoms she had experienced, and no one could diagnose, were typical for the disease. She also learned that the disease was called lupus (the wolf) because it can attack anywhere. The problems Crystal encountered, all came to mind:

- Kidney problems and infections
- Muscle lumps that come and go
- Inflamed joints that seem to come and go
- Headaches that make you want to die
- Voice problems due to inflammation in her voice box
- Fatigue that drugs, coffee, and candy make worse

As its final statement, the Lupus Foundation said: "It's a fatal illness." Great! She could expect to die from lupus.

By December of 1981, Crystal was in so much pain she called her husband to her bedside and put her physical condition in two words: "I'm dying." Her husband's reaction was, "No way!" He called the Shaklee distributor because he had heard some tapes that said good nutrition seemed to help people with lupus. At least they felt better.

Her initial nutrition program included Instant Protein, which made her gag, Vita-lea, which gave her a queasy stomach, Vita-C, B-Complex, and up to seven Herb-Lax a day to start. She noticed two things: protein gave her energy, and Herb-Lax gave her regularity. This proves she reacts normally to some things.

After a few week she noticed that she was not only regular, but was taking only one daily nap in the afternoon. Besides that, she was doing more of the cleaning and daily household chores rather than just sitting around. She felt better than she had ever felt. After listening to some tapes on nutrition, she became so motivated, that she told the doctor she was going off the drugs. He laughed and said, "Okay, but let's do it slowly." She did it gradually and, much to his surprise, succeeded.

About two years later, during a particularly stressful time, Crystal had a flare-up of the lupus, along with some typical female problems that necessitated surgery. In spite of telling the doctor she didn't want any more steroids, she woke up from the surgery and was put on 40 milligrams of Prednisone daily. Crystal felt she was starting all over again. But this time she had built her reserves with a good nutrition program and, with the doctor's help, got off Prednisone once again.

Unfortunately, lupus waited a couple more years and attacked her kidneys. Kidney problems are not minor league; they're always serious. You can't live without working kidneys. Consequently, Crystal required medication to keep her kidneys working, but by sticking with her good diet and supplement program, she was soon able to get off that medication as well.

About this time Crystal was regularly listening to tapes on nutrition, and began to develop a Shaklee business. At first it paid for her prodigious product use, but she also saw people get results and started to feel the joy that comes to people who help others. As she got more into her business, she started listening to motivational tapes, which started her on the road to positive thinking. Pretty soon she was attending motivational seminars by such leaders as Nevena Christi and Rick Hill. Her life changed. Besides feeling good about herself, her family, and the world, she had also found satisfaction.

A year ago she went for a complete checkup by a specialist in rheumatology. He gave her a thorough evaluation, including blood tests, x-rays, and everything he could think of that might be relevant. First he told her she didn't look her age, 60. Then he said the best words of all: "I can't find any evidence of lupus right now." But Crystal knows, and all the experts confirm, that the lupus is simply sleeping. Like its name suggests, it will attack if she provokes it and lets her guard down for an instant.

Her "guard" includes an excellent diet that is based on the following:

- No red meat
- No sugar or white flour
- Lots of cranberry juice
- No dairy products
- Foods that cause a flare-up for her are avoided. These include citrus fruits.
- A supplement program that includes Instant Protein, Vita Lea, Vita-C, B-Complex, EPA, vitamin E, and alfalfa tablets.

Stress control is also part of her "guard," along with a good nutrition program that gives her body a strong foundation, so all its needs are met. Along with nutrition, stress control calls for a positive outlook and the ability to let problems roll off you, like water off a duck's back. Crystal has become a positive woman who radiates good cheer and self confidence.

IS THIS IN CRYSTAL'S HEAD?

No way! About 85 percent of lupus victims are women. It's inherited and often passed to men by their mothers. Crystal's story is quite typical.

It's not uncommon for victims of lupus to bounce from one doctor to another without a diagnosis, just as Crystal had done. Often the diagnosis will include kidney infection, the result of food poisoning, or a lingering systemic infection. Only after everything seems to be ruled out, lupus is diagnosed. In 1992, it's not as confusing as it was in 1962.

It's typical for the victim to be tired. This tiredness isn't relieved by either a good night's sleep or naps during the day. It's as if the body can't get its energy back.

WHAT DOES NUTRITION DO FOR LUPUS?

A chronic illness produces many side effects that can be overcome by a good diet and good nutrition. Having irregular bowel movements and being tired are typical.

The lack of a bowel movement every 36 hours or less

is usually indicative of a poor diet. Recall how Crystal drifted to eating lots of processed foods, especially candy. Many drugs, including steroids, often cause constipation or make it worse. Consequently, the Herb-Lax helped to make her regular again.

Regularity helped her body eliminate the same toxins that kept a flare-up going. Add Alfalfa, and you increase a special type of fiber that is especially good at binding the materials excreted through the gall bladder. So, Herb-Lax and alfalfa worked together to bring on regularity and eliminate toxins.

Instant Protein, though Crystal didn't like it at first, was the best energy source she could use. Instant Protein provides sustained energy without calling on the body to produce insulin. When insulin is put into the blood, it causes blood sugar to drop. When blood sugar drops, it leads to the desire for more sugar, usually in the form of candy. Candy quickly elevates blood sugar and makes you sleepy. Sound like Crystal's symptoms? By using Instant Protein, she eliminated all those complexities and had a good sustained-energy source.

Her supplement program was excellent. A body under the stress of a a chronic illness needs more nourishment. One added benefit of Crystal's program is the EPA. EPA helps shift the body's metabolic processes in favor of the prostaglandins that modulate and reduce inflammation.

An additional benefit is the elimination of headaches. These headaches seem to be part of the inflammatory symptoms. In some clinical studies, EPA was shown to be effective in reducing and eliminating headaches.

Finally, Crystal noticed that by using lots of cranberry juice, she eliminated bladder infections. This practice goes back to Finnish folklore as a therapeutic or preventive side-effect of cloudberries. Cloudberries are similar to cranberries, although they are yellow in color. Clinical research has proven that a substance in the juice of these berries prevents bacteria from holding on to the bladder membranes. If the bacteria can't attach, the infection can't get started or keep going. So, using cranberry juice regularly eliminates many bladder infections, and is a common preventive program for people confined to wheelchairs.

WILL NUTRITION CURE LUPUS?

Absolutely not! But it can make life much better. Any chronic illness is a constant stress on the body and causes all of the body's systems to be vulnerable. No one really knows what a chronically ill body requires.

Nutritional needs are unknown because it would be almost impossible to do the right nutrient-balance studies. When a person is chronically ill, you can't ask them to volunteer for additional research, so the only recourse is to increase their nutrition program sensibly and observe. In most cases, positive nutrition produces an improvement in health.

A POSITIVE OUTLOOK

Crystal noticed that she felt better when she worked her Shaklee business, and when she attended motivational seminars. This wonderful response falls into the category I call "positive outlook."

A Shaklee direct-selling business can't be built without a positive outlook. You have to see the good side of things. A "no" isn't a negative to you; it's a person depriving themselves of an opportunity. Motivational seminars are dripping with positive energy. A good leader guides you to acquiring a positive outlook.

People with a positive outlook live longer. In a clinic study, Stanford Medical School divided terminally ill people with cancer into two groups. One was given regular, motivational programs by an experienced leader. The other group was given books to read on a positive outlook, without the guidance of a leader. The people with the motivated leader lived 18 months longer, on average.

Similar studies have been conducted to show that an optimistic outlook improves sleep, energy, work efficiency, and family life. Crystal's experience was typical. As an aside, young people with an optimistic outlook are likely to not use drugs or get into trouble.

CHAPTER
15 Macular Degeneration

JEYTON'S STORY

When Jeyton couldn't focus on street signs and house numbers, people said, "it's aging." Any glare became very uncomfortable and her eyes hurt. Then she started noticing gray, shadowy areas while she was reading. After reading for a short time, her eyes felt strained. In the morning her eyelids stuck shut. Eventually, small ulcers developed on her eyeballs. In 1982, these painful ulcers led to a complete eye examination, which produced a short, two-word diagnosis: macular degeneration. Put another way: You're going blind!

WHAT IS MACULAR DEGENERATION?

A small area, less than 1/4 inch on the retina of the eye, where central vision and color perception takes place, is named the macula. The macula is essential for focusing the eye. It makes it possible to read, see detail, and focus on close or distant objects. For example, you can read this page, say ten inches away, and then focus on a star a million light years away in an instant. If the macula fails, you can't focus, everything is a blur, and you're left with only the ability to see light and dark. A little peripheral vision sometimes remains, but not enough to stop you from being declared "legally blind."

When this peripheral vision survives after the macula is gone, a set of binocular-like devices can be prescribed to help you get around. The binocular device is difficult to wear and isn't much help, but it's better than no vision at all. However, it lets the person function without a seeing-eye dog.

As we age, the blood vessels that supply the macula often harden. When the blood flow declines, the cells that form the macula begin to die and central vision deteriorates. Your ability to read normal print goes first and eventually all central vision disappears. As the macula degenerates, it progresses from a soft, delicate, depressed area on the retina, to a raised hard bump. About 16,000 new cases of blindness occur each year from macular degeneration. That's almost two people every hour, 24 hours a day.

Macular degeneration has always been considered an age-related form of blindness. It parallels general hardening of the arteries, which usually progresses as we get older. Most research efforts were directed toward helping the victim use the peripheral vision that remained. This meant the development of various optical devices and special large-print books. Few scientists looked for either a cure or, more importantly, a preventive approach. Don't get the impression from this that research scientists and physicians are close minded. The issue here is the terminology "it's part of aging." Whenever an illness gets labeled that way, the door on research is usually shut. After all, why investigate something that's simply part of being normal?

BACK TO JEYTON

In February 1984, Jeyton sought a second opinion from a specialist in the closest city, Corpus Christi, Texas. Diagnosis: macular degeneration! The doctor could give no encouragement for her visual future and offered literature that taught victims of macular degeneration how to cope, while becoming blind in slow motion. His recommendation was to learn how to live as a blind person, while she could still see.

After the 1984 diagnosis, Jeyton tried to carry on life as usual. She didn't complain nor burden her family or friends. As her vision deteriorated, she got stronger and stronger prescription glasses. Since street signs became fuzzy and she lost the ability to focus, she drove less and less. She had become resigned to the diagnosis, so she sought understanding from literature and organizations dedicated to macular degeneration. Since macular degeneration has already claimed over 240,000 eyes, the organization has lots of members and it's growing.

Jeyton's most depressing experience was when she attended the February 1988 convention for people with macular degeneration. Experts at the convention said there was no cure. Support people showed various optical devices to help victims of the disease cope with life. In her words, "I was profoundly discouraged. They wouldn't give the slightest glimmer of hope for a cure. We were treated as if our vision was lost." But in spite of experiencing her slow loss of sight, Jeyton couldn't simply give up. She couldn't visualize herself as blind.

Later, in the same spring of 1988, Jeyton was watching the evening news when a doctor being interviewed told how some people with macular degeneration were helped with zinc. Shortly after that, an article appeared in *Readers' Digest* telling about research conducted by Dr. David A. Newsome of the Louisiana State University Eye Center. Newsome's research showed that the development of macular degeneration could be slowed by taking 200 milligrams of zinc daily. In his study, the volunteers got 100 milligrams of zinc twice daily or a placebo. Of those who got the zinc, the degeneration slowed or even stopped.

By now, Jeyton's vision had deteriorated to 20/40. This meant she could focus on things very close, but things at even a short distance were fuzzy at best and most often a blur. She decided that was as bad as she would ever let it get. She was going to start a program of zinc supplements. Jeyton adjusted her Shaklee supplement-program to include 200 milligrams of zinc. She kept a daily scorecard so that whatever supplements she used, they included 200 milligrams of zinc.

By November 1988, five months later, her eye doctor said the macula in each eye had improved. Improvement means the area of the macula looked softer and not raised; it was closer to normal. This was confirmed by a quantitative test, which showed vision of 20/30, an easily correctable nearsightedness. This meant that the eye doctor's subjective conclusion was confirmed by the tests.

In December 1989, eighteen months after starting her

zinc regimen, her left eye showed no macular degeneration. Her right eye had just a slight indication of degeneration and tested at 20/25, which is very close to normal. With 20/25 vision, you don't need glasses.

By January 1991, the disease was completely eliminated. Her vision tests at 20/20 in both eyes and there is no visual evidence of macular degeneration. Jeyton is cured.

THE CURE

Was It in Her Head?

No, it was in her eyeballs. The retina of the eye is really an extension of the brain, and is one of the last frontiers of nutritional biochemistry research. For example, eye tissues, including the retina, contain many nutrients in concentrations 50 to 100 times of that found in the blood that bathes them. This means that those tissues must expend energy to concentrate these nutrients. It's like pumping water up from a deep well. If you need the water, you pump. Usually there is no problem for the tissue to concentrate these nutrients, and all that's required of us is to achieve the Recommended Daily Allowance (RDA) of most nutrients. But what happens if something goes wrong with the system that extracts the nutrients from our blood, or the system that builds the nutrient in the tissues isn't working? We've got to give them some help. In fact, lots of help. Help under these conditions means getting much more zinc than the RDA. Chemists would call this applying the law of mass action. If you use the well analogy, it's like raising the water table so you don't need to pump as hard.

Two-hundred milligrams of zinc daily is over 10 times the RDA for zinc. At that level, eye tissues could get the zinc, but it still took almost two years for Jeyton's eyes to return to normal. That's what I mean when I say nutrition works in slow motion.

Loss of visual sensitivity, which is another type of retinal degeneration that involves vitamin E, was recently reversed with vitamin-E supplements at a level even higher than 10 times the RDA. But it took two years for complete reversal. This time frame is similar to Jeyton's experience with zinc. Both eye conditions confirm that people aren't all the same, and some require more than the RDA of certain nutrients to stay healthy. More importantly, it serves notice on people who expect nutrition to produce fast results like modern miracle drugs. Nutrition doesn't work that way; it takes time.

Is zinc a drug in Jeyton's case? I don't think so. Obviously, Jeyton was not zinc deficient by the classical definition of zinc deficiency. She didn't have acne nor the taste and smell aberrations that come with zinc deficiency, her energy level was high, her cuts healed correctly, she followed a good diet, and had always taken Shaklee Vita-Lea. Since Vita-Lea provides the RDA for zinc (18 milligrams), Jeyton had always achieved her RDA even if her diet slipped. In short, she had practiced sensible supplementation and nutrition insurance. But the zinc RDA set for normal people simply wasn't enough for Jeyton.

Suppose, in her case, we take a healthy macula as a criterion of adequate nutrition. Then you'd have to agree that she was deficient and needed more zinc. Jeyton's zinc RDA is not 15 milligrams, it's higher; possibly as high as

200 milligrams. Do you think anyone with macular degeneration wants to test for exactly how much zinc they need? I doubt it. Taking 200 milligrams is harmless, so why not?

Jeyton's zinc requirement is not easily determined, but by taking the amount she does, she has her sight. It's important to understand that drugs can *not* be used in the same way. Everyone requires zinc to live. Some people require a drug to cure an illness, so they can live as near to normal a life as possible. There's a world of difference between zinc requirements and drugs. Drugs are prescribed by doctors for a specific purpose and should be taken as directed. All drugs have side effects, and misuse can be devastating, if not fatal. At 200-milligrams daily, zinc has no noticeable side-effects.

16 Mental Development: From Last to First

STEVEN'S STORY

Geri had her worst nightmare when she was wide awake. "A significant part of your son's brain is very poorly developed. He will never be able to learn, may never walk, and will always require custodial care." The pediatric neurologist was compassionate and polite, but his words cut into her like a red-hot poker. Geri was devastated.

At the time, Geri and Lindy had two teenaged daughters and a son Steven, aged two. They were supportive parents and super achievers. Geri taught gifted children English in grades seven through nine, and had built a small jewelry business, specializing in diamonds, as her spare-time occupation. Lindy, a graphic artist, had built his own successful graphic-arts business. Both daughters were bright and did well in school. The girls were self reliant, active in school, full of fun, and close to each other. Steven came along when the youngest daughter was nine.

Steven wasn't growing well; the family could see that

themselves. Any child, including an Asian-Hawaiian child, should weigh double Steven's 19 pounds at two-years-old. "We all knew things weren't going well, but we had hope with a dash of denial thrown in. At age two, Steven could only drag himself around and make some noises," Lindy said, and then continued. "It was very depressing. The pediatrician had recommended him for the state tests, so we would know how much we could expect of him. In retrospect, the doctor was also helping us to face the situation more fully."

I.Q. tests are done by expert pediatric-neurologists. Although difficult to conduct at age two, Steven came in with a score of 50. Geri's professional education gave her a good understanding of these tests and she knew that, at best, the tests were off by ten points, so his I.Q. could also be 40 or 60. She knew from listening to the experts, that the most they could ever hope for was a ten-point gain; so, Steven's maximum IQ would be about 70 if everything went his way. A pretty bleak outlook by any standards. He could be trained, for instance, to polish cars or clean buildings, but that was about the extent of what they could hope for him.

"I was depressed all the time and cried a lot," Geri said. "I'd be driving along and just start crying without even thinking about it. One day our daughter Terri changed things. She said, 'Mom, you can't let them put Steven in a box at two-years-old. There's got to be more in his life than that. We must pull together and bring him along.' " Terri's optimism picked up Geri's spirits, but she still didn't know what to do.

Steven was receiving help from two experts: a physical therapist to help him use his muscles, and a speech therapist to try and develop his vocal capacity. Both were polite to Geri, but never very enthusiastic about Steven's progress.

The supervising pediatrician called on a nutritionist to help improve Steven's growth, as he was so small for his age. Steven would only drink his milk from a baby bottle—seven bottles a day! Both the doctor and nutritionist told Geri to feed him table food. What does table food mean when everyone is eating separately?

Geri asked the pediatrician if Steven was getting adequate nutrition from the milk. She laughed as she told me his reply: "Milk is nature's complete food, so it's all right." The pediatrician went further and told her not to bother with the baby vitamins any longer, because the amount of milk he was drinking would give him everything he needed. "The nutritionist confirmed all this, so I was confident," she said.

Geri was certain she was doing all she could for Steven, but was always looking for more. Her friends and colleagues were considerate and supportive. "When Steven was sitting in my office, they would say, 'Oh, what a well-behaved child'." She continued, "I wanted to hear, 'Oh, what a bright, active child'. But everyone was trying to be complimentary and help us along. I'm thankful for that."

A close friend asked Geri to attend a nutrition luncheon one Saturday. The speaker was Barbara Lagoni, a dietician, who was speaking on nutrition in general, and Shaklee products in particular. The friend told Geri she'd be able to get good answers from Barb.

"I didn't really have the time to go to this meeting, and knew I could see the staff nutritionist any time I wanted by just asking the pediatrician, but something in my subconscious told me to go." After the meeting, where Barbara discussed the need for protein and supplements, a question came to Geri's mind, but her Asian politeness kept her from asking it in public. So she tried to talk to Barb after the meeting was over.

"Although the speaker was mobbed after the meeting, a path cleared for me, and I got to ask her my question: Is milk really a complete food for my child?" Geri briefly explained Steven's situation. Barbara, clearly taken by the situation, gave the right answer in a very gentle way: "Nowadays, we realize that cow's milk can't possibly provide every thing a child of two years requires. There are too many critical nutrients missing." The answer, though short, gave Geri lots of food for thought.

That very night Geri purchased some Shaklee products and added protein and vitamins to Steven's milk. She pricked open lecithin and EPA, ground up Vita-Lea by putting it in a handkerchief and pounding it with a hammer, and stirred the mix into Steven's milk. Steven had no trouble drinking the nutrition-laced milk. In fact, he liked the protein flavor. "Now, looking back, it must have been a welcome change for him." She laughed and said, "Anything would probably taste good after seven bottles of plain milk."

Lindy proudly explained the results: "Within about two weeks we could see brightness in Steven's eyes, although we were hoping it wasn't in our minds. Up until then, his eyes were dull and not bright. They now took on a sparkle. After three months on the nutrition milk, as we called it, we had no doubts. Steven was definitely more alert. The girls could see it when they played with him. He wasn't dragging; he was trying to crawl. He acted curious and would look at things as if he was studying them. We knew the nutrition was doing something positive, as well as the physical and speech therapy. The therapists also seemed to have become more interested in Steven."

Six months after starting the Shaklee program, the physical therapist said Steven was progressing much more rapidly than she had ever expected. She thought Steven would not go far, but said he was showing good progress.

The speech therapist noticed some coherence and direction to his sound and observed more progress than his tests predicted. She said that Steven was trying to use his tongue to make sounds, which was far more than they expected him to try. Geri told the therapists she felt the nutrition was definitely doing something and was helping Steven respond to their efforts better. "I got a polite smile from each therapist." She laughs now, in retrospect.

By this time, Steven was three and time to be tested again. These tests are administered annually to children, like Steven, by pediatric neurologists who specialize in child development. They carefully use the same tests and testing methods, so they can compare each child to thousands of other children with similar disabilities and in similar programs. After the test is scored and reviewed by a panel of experts, they can see how rapidly the child learns. This way, progress or the lack of it is not the figment of someone's imagination.

When Steven's rate of learning tapers off, the tests will show his decline early enough so his therapist won't frustrate him by pushing too hard. The testing allows Steven to develop to his potential and not aim for some arbitrary standard. Everyone wins when this system is used correctly.

Geri watched through a one-way mirror as Steven was given the 20-minute test by the pediatrician. "The doctor would work with Steven for a few minutes and then go to her desk for a different test. She did this four times. Finally, in an hour and a half, she finished. Steven didn't seem tired; in fact he seemed to enjoy the testing. I didn't know whether to be scared or happy. I was all nerves."

The doctor couldn't believe it was the same child. She was so enthusiastic about Steven that she walked Geri to the elevator and said: "We have to compile all the scores and you'll have the results in about three days."

The reason the doctor kept getting new tests was because the tests for retarded children didn't apply to Steven any longer. She kept trying slightly more advanced tests until she wound up using the test for normal children. The doctor realized that even though Steven couldn't speak, he could follow verbal instructions. The experts estimated his I.Q. at 103 to 106, based on these tests. Even with the ten point error range, this finding put Steven in the normal range! They could drop car polishing as his profession.

Lindy continues the story with a gleam in his eye. "Things had become very different at home. Steven had stopped dragging and started crawling. He was full of energy and had lots of stamina. At 37 pounds, he was now in the normal weight range for a three-year-old. His muscles had developed some tone, so his arms and legs took on form. He could actually get out a few words."

Steven was given exactly the same test program when he was four-years-old. These rigorously applied tests monitor his progress and continue to compare him to thousands of children. At this stage, his tests indicated he was progressing normally for his age.

Steven was put in a program for normal children. He now speaks in sentences of seven to ten words and uses pronouns. He can express abstract thoughts, which is a sure sign of a normal I.Q. Remember, intelligence is the ability to integrate information from diverse sources. That's what Steven was doing at that point.

At age four, Steven used a small walker to help himself get around, but most of the time at home, he stands and walks unassisted. With his normal I.Q., and continuing physical development, he'll be entering school along with children his own age. He'll be in a normal classroom with normal children.

Steven continues his nutrition program. His protein goes into his orange juice, which he swirls to keep it from settling out. His supplements consist of children's Vita-Lea, lecithin, and EPA. Sometimes he takes more, but this group is his basic standby.

WHOSE HEAD IS IT IN?

Steven's story depicts the strength of the human spirit. Give the body the right nourishment, and it will develop to its maximum potential. Nourishment, however, begins with the nutrients: protein, vitamins, and minerals. How fortunate that Geri went to Barbara Lagoni's seminar. Nourishment must also include nurturing by loving, caring, and supportive people. Steven had that in abundance.

I think his older sister stated it very clearly when she said to her mother, "Don't let Steven be boxed in. No one knows what his life will be like. He has human spirit just like all of us, and no one can stop that."

SOME THOUGHTS

People can overcome many handicaps, as the brain has incredible recuperative powers. This story doesn't say, that with a little protein, the undeveloped part of Steven's brain developed all at once in a year. More likely, other parts of his brain took over for the undeveloped part or helped compensate for what that part should do. However, the development couldn't have happened as well, if at all, without the correct nourishment.

In recent years, research has shown that essential oils from lecithin and EPA are required for mental development. Indeed, papers have appeared in the medical journals that show children who don't get these oils are behind in their mental development. Some papers even suggest that these children have a deficiency. This trend indicates that these oils will achieve a much higher status in the future.

Does Steven require more of these oils than average? I don't know, but neither does anyone else, and it will be decades before researchers find out. In addition, some parts of the brain can use amino acids for nourishment. This has been proven time and again and Instant Protein, as well as milk, has amino acids. Therefore, did Steven's brain require more than it could get from milk and normal food? I'll bet it did. If his body didn't develop correctly, whose to say his digestive-absorptive system was spared? Without these organs working correctly, he couldn't be getting enough nourishment.

Is it in the heads of Geri and Lindy? If it is, you'd have to explain away to the experts who tested Steven, as well as the physical and speech therapists. Steven's now a normal young boy developing along with the rest of the kids his age.

17 Migraine Headache

ROSANNA'S STORY

"I was 15 when I got my first migraine headache. It was like living out my worst nightmare. The headache would start over my left eye, spread to my temple in about an hour or two, and in six hours it would reach my neck. Once the headache got to the base of my head, there was no stopping it."

Experience taught Rosanna that the six hours it took for the headache to progress from just over her left eye to the base of her neck, were all the time she had left to get things done. In her words, "Whatever I had to do, I had only six hours to do it in, because I spent the next one- to three-days away from the human race, in hell."

"Experience taught me that once the headache started, there was one thing to do: lie totally still on my back in a dark room, until the headache went away. If I lifted my head or even rolled over, severe nausea would come over me. At that point, the only relief I could think of was death." Her description goes on. "Any noise hurt so much that no torture devised by man could be worse."

MIGRAINE: A MODERN FRONTIER

Every day you can witness miracles in any modern hospital. Kidney transplants have become routine; heart, lung and liver transplants are regular procedures; and as I write this, over ten complete intestinal tracts have been transplanted in Pittsburg alone. A quintuple by-pass — that's five arteries transplanted — is so routine, it's not treated as special. Over 90 percent of people who undergo such spectacular surgery recover from the surgery. Think of it like this: Suppose you had been a professor of medicine at Harvard Medical School in 1900 and died at that time. Then, suppose you could somehow return to watch these medical procedures take place today. Many of them would seem almost magical. They would compare in outcome to the miracles in the New Testament. Infections that, in 1900, had been fatal and without hope, are now routinely knocked out with an antibiotic. Instead of dying, the patient goes back to work in a few days. What you then knew as a hopelessly demented person confined to an institution, now only needs to take a drug twice daily and they look, act, and work like any normal person. There are many of these people in all walks of life.

However, in spite of these miraculous accomplishments, we still can't eliminate migraine headaches. This seems incongruous in comparison to the miracles of surgery, and our ability to defeat infection, control high blood pressure, and manic depression. After all, a headache, even a migraine headache, seems mundane compared to these other illnesses. But that's how it is with migraines. There's a lot of help available for its victims, but most of the help deals with fighting its symptoms and not stopping the cause.

WHAT'S A MIGRAINE?

Rosanna described it in her own words, as well as any medical manual could. "A migraine usually starts around the eye and progresses in three- to six-hours to the entire head, down to the neck. Once established over the head, the headache lasts 24 to 72 hours. A migraine can include nausea and sometimes vomiting, but the nausea is severe and vomiting isn't a relief like in stomach upset. A migraine sufferer naturally seeks seclusion while the headache is in progress and usually learns, on their own, to lie completely still in a dark, quiet room until the headache goes away. If it lasts three days, that means three days in a noiseless, dark room!"

Migraine headaches are caused by a disturbance of cranial circulation. In other words, circulation in the skull is disturbed. Blood vessels in the scalp dilate and they cause the generalized head pain. Since nausea occurs with the slightest movement, you can guess that the inner-ear balance center is either directly or indirectly involved.

While nausea is a routine symptom, other symptoms are not consistent. Migraine sufferers often see flashes of light, and straight lines will appear wavy. So the visual centers are also involved. Hands and feet often become cold and the victim will feel chilled, even in warm weather. Many migraine sufferers become hypersensitive to the slightest noise that most of us wouldn't even notice. Noise becomes an extremely painful event for them.

Of the eight-million migraine sufferers in the United States, three times as many of them are women as men. Over 50 percent of people, men or women, who get migraines, have a family history of them (usually a parent). Consequently, there's a genetic predisposition to migraines, even if they aren't absolutely inherited. Of women who get them, over 60 percent relate them to their menstrual cycle. This means that they often precede menses. These women are also likely to have irregular periods. However, the migraines are not confined to the menstrual cycle. It's just the most likely time for them to occur.

Of the 60 percent of women who relate migraines to their menstrual cycle, most of them noticed that their migraines don't occur during pregnancy. This observation, and the fact that the migraines disappear altogether around menopause, suggests a strong hormonal relationship. Some researchers believe that drastic changes in hormonal balance cause these women to get migraines. In other words, it's not the absolute levels of hormones; it's the balance of one to the other. This also invokes stress as a factor, because these hormonal changes are a severe stress on the body.

Women who get migraines usually grow out of them by about the age of 50, during menopause. This signals a hormonal involvement. As you read on, you'll see that there is some evidence that migraines act like an inflammatory illness in some people. If it is inflammatory, it's reasonable to expect a hormonal involvement, similar to rheumatoid arthritis.

Other recent research strongly suggests that some migraines are an inflammatory disease. You could think of them as a form of arthritis. For this reason, anti-inflammatory drugs, such as Ponstel, that inhibit prostaglandin PGE_2, bring some relief. Other research shows that EPA causes the body to produce prostaglandin PGE_3, which helps relieve migraines. PGE_2 aggravates inflammation, and PGE_3 modulates it.

Folklore had taught that an herb, feverfew, relieved migraine headaches. An English medical group conducted a clinical study and confirmed the folk wisdom. This finding supports the inflammatory nature, because feverfew interferes with the body's production of PGE_2.

In support of the inflammatory nature of migraines, research in England, Italy, the United States, and a few other countries has shown that migraines are triggered in some people by selective foods. Foods that consistently trigger migraines are chocolate, cheese, and those rich in monosodium glutamate, MSG. Red wine also initiates migraines. However, not all migraines are triggered by food or wine. All people recognize stress as a cause of migraines, so both observations, food and stress, fit the inflammatory pattern very well.

So, although the cause of migraines is unknown, both personal experience and research point to the pattern of an inflammatory disease. Even if the cause of migraines is unknown, much of the statistics suggest a dietary, stress-related, hormonal-balance pattern. One thing is certain, when a migraine comes on, it's terrible. Let me return to Rosanna.

BACK TO ROSANNA

Rosanna's mother had suffered from migraines, albeit not as severely as Rosanna. Consequently, Rosanna searched for a doctor who could treat her for them even if they couldn't make them go away. Like most migraine sufferers, she went to any doctor she thought could help, including medical doctors who specialized in neurologic disorders, chiropractors, osteopaths, and others.

Depending on the doctor's specialty, she was told that her migraines were caused by her menstrual cycle, because she was irregular; heredity, because her mother had them; and the permanent stress from an auto accident she had at age 19, even if the accident occured four years after her first migraine started.

Rosanna's parents sent her to a pain clinic in Michigan. Here she learned how to live with migraines and why she must lie still in a quiet and dark place while going through the attack. She tried yoga, physical therapy, and anything she thought would help. Rosanna's experience proves the observation, quite clearly, that, after all is said and done, migraine sufferers are really on their own.

By noting when, how, and under what circumstances the migraines started, Rosanna learned that hers could be caused by stress, either good or bad. In other words, an uplifting, happy day could bring one on as well as a bad, tension-filled day. Other things that triggered the migraines were: a major shift in the weather pattern, when the barometric pressure changes dramatically; a day filled with taxing mental or physical work; a chill, especially on her neck where she was hurt in the auto accident; too much sun; fumes from automobile exhaust, such as during a bad traffic tie-up.

As an aside, all these environmental triggers indicate an inflammatory pattern. The neck injury is similar to the person with rheumatoid arthritis who had an old joint injury. It all fits. Rosanna could protect herself from most of these things. For example, wear a scarf around her neck, have her auto gas pumped by an attendant, be sure to go easy with physical work, and don't get too enthusiastic or overly involved in group activities. Rosanna was also careful to avoid the foods that trigger migraines. However, some things were unavoidable like her period, changes in the weather, some foods, and an occasional bad day.

A big step to deal with emotionally was getting married. She and her husband-to-be prepared the wedding very carefully and proved what determined people can accomplish if they really try. They selected a wedding date that she felt would fall between migraines and then deliberately planned everything, so as the wedding date approached, nothing would surface unexpectedly. This planning avoided the stress normally associated with weddings. It worked. Rosanna made it through the wedding and honeymoon without a migraine. This is proof of how well she had learned to schedule her life around this terrible affliction and handle situations that arose.

Rosanna and her husband were blessed with two children. Not only did Rosanna experience the joy of motherhood, but pregnancy brought complete freedom from migraines. In her own words: "I asked myself, are they over for good?" Within 30-days after she stopped nursing the baby, a migraine reared its ugly head. She said it nicely: "I realized I couldn't always be pregnant or nursing, but it was nice to have the relief for awhile."

Her obstetrician was impressed by her pregnancy experience, so he tried giving her a drug he used for women with another disorder, endometriosis. Unfortunately, the drug didn't work, but her doctor's intentions were good and he, at least, could put one idea to rest.

Although Rosanna and her husband had learned to live with her migraines and were doing fine at raising two children, the migraines were a terrible drag. They were like a spectre hanging over everything they did and required careful thought and planning for even the slightest outing. For this reason, they never stopped searching for some way to prevent the migraines.

Both Rosanna and her husband attended many seminars. At one nutrition seminar a Shaklee distributor spoke of a migraine sufferer who had been helped by nutritional supplements. About two weeks after the seminar, Rosanna got a real bad 72-hour migraine. Her husband called the Shaklee distributor and said: "We want to try some products."

She started with a modest program that included Instant Protein, Vita-Lea, B-Complex, EPA, and Herb-Lax. Just eight days later, they got bad news and good news. The bad news: Rosanna got a migraine. The good news: It lasted only two and a half hours! If this relief was going to last, it sounded too easy. Her first thought was that it was in her head. She would gladly settle for a severe two and a half hour headache every eight to ten days. For Rosanna, that would be miraculous. Her husband wouldn't let her back down on the program. He kept her going to see what would evolve.

Another part of Rosanna's story is constipation. It cleared up when she started her Shaklee program. Since Rosanna started her program, she has spoken to many groups of migraine sufferers and noticed that most of them have bowel irregularity in the form of constipation. One can speculate on how constipation could aggravate a migraine in the same way it aggravates asthma. Hopefully, researchers will shed more light on this relationship in the future.

Rosanna related the following story: "I kept the program going. I mixed Meal Shakes with Instant Protein and increased all my supplements. I waited 30 days, two months, then ten months. No more migraines! This was a miracle to me."

It's now been over four years since Rosanna has had a migraine. She's careful not to get chills, manages the external stress in her life, and doesn't overwork and get tired. As an Italian, she still loves some provolone cheese now and then, but she otherwise follows a strict nutrition program which includes four basic supplements: B-Complex, EPA, calcium-magnesium, and alfalfa. She also uses Vita-Lea, Vita-C, and other products, but the big four are her basics.

If she feels a headache starting, she doubles or even triples up on the big four. Around her periods, which are irregular and are preceded by two days of cramping, she routinely doubles up on her supplements without even thinking about it. Her commitment to a careful lifestyle and this nutrition program prevents the headache from starting.

Ask Rosanna if she feels she has found a cure and you'll get a surprising answer. "No! I'll always be a migraine sufferer." This plan isn't a cure; it's only what it takes to prevent them from getting started. At her request, the gynecologist, who helped her as much as he could, gave her a thorough examination. He also did a complete review of her medical history, including the migraines, once again.

His conclusion: "Keep up what you're doing. It's drug free and it works. We don't have a better plan."

IS IT IN HER HEAD?

I guess migraines are always in your head, but Rosanna has learned how to keep them out of her head. Her program, even though she came upon it by trial and error, makes scientific sense. B-Complex in large doses helps to improve circulation to the extremities, including the head. Most folks who don't get migraines observe this circulation effect as improved fingernail growth. EPA helps increase the body's production of prostaglandin PGE3. This prostaglandin reduces an inflammatory response. This effect has been confirmed in a number of excellent clinical studies. EPA forms the basis of a previous book I wrote entitled *The Arthritis Relief Diet*. This diet is a plan to reduce inflammation, because a complete diet with supplements is far more powerful than supplements alone.

Alfalfa helps reduce Rosanna's sinus congestion, which is another inflammatory response. The fiber in alfalfa, specifically the saponins in the fiber, bind antagonists produced in the liver and excreted through the gall bladder. Saponins remove them where they enter the gastrointestinal tract, so they're eliminated totally. As a woman, Rosanna needs more calcium, and there have been hypotheses that migraines can even be precipitated by inadequate magnesium.

Magnesium is a nutrient, usually short in the diet, that has a very important role in health. I like to say it's an "unsung hero." Other supplements Rosanna uses simply improve her general health. And the healthier her body is, the better it will deal with stress, whether it be physical or mental.

PHYLLIS

"You say a broken back was a blessing in disguise?" I asked. "Look," she continued, "you don't need to be smart all your life. Just once will do." Phyllis' life had been miserable until shortly after that fateful day when she was hit by a New Orleans' streetcar. I'd better digress a little.

Phyllis lived in New Orleans. She was troubled with migraine headaches about twice a month and couldn't eat when she had them. In fact, she represents another group of migraine sufferers: those who become somewhat anorexigenic. They aren't necessarily anorexigenic people, it's just that the migraines seem to start them in that direction. Perhaps the intense nausea that comes with migraines, or the recognition, even subconsciously, that some foods trigger the headaches, causes these people to become anorexigenic. You don't need a degree in clinical psychology to see that either nausea or the idea that food causes migraines could create an aversion to food. Just reread how Rosanna described the headaches.

So besides the migraines, poor nutrition started taking its toll on Phyllis' life. She had gingivitis. If she sank her teeth into anything solid, her gums started bleeding. In addition, her teeth were loose. In short, she was not a very healthy or physically-fit person. If you saw her, then you'd probably say she was "sickly."

When Phyllis was hit by a car, it was one more turn in the downward spiral of her life. She didn't have to go far from the broken back to find a bottom in her life. While she was in the hospital, a friend asked her to try Shaklee products. Her friend knew she ate poorly and wanted her to heal as quickly as possible. Fortunately, the broken back wasn't a crippling type, but it still needed to heal. There was a 30-day guarantee on the products, and her life couldn't get worse, so she started on a program like Rosanna's.

In six weeks she was out of the hospital. Phyllis had re-covered from a broken back in record time. Her gums had healed and didn't bleed anymore. She could even eat hospital food. "Then it dawned on me what had really hap-pened. The migraines were gone. I started life all over again. I was given a second chance."

Phyllis started a Shaklee business. One of her first deci-sions was to have her teeth capped once the business start-ed paying. Now that her gums had healed, she knew she'd keep her teeth, so why not get them fixed? And by the way, she's had no more migraines.

ONE, LAST OBSERVATION

Phyllis is one of many stories of how migraine headaches often clear up with a good nutrition program. Though her gingivitis seems like a little icing on the cake, it's not. Recent research at Tufts' Medical School showed quite clearly that some people who have chronic gingivitis can clear it completely with about 600-milligrams daily of vitamin C. So while Phyllis proved the power of good nutrition, she also confirmed that each of us is an in-dividual with our own nutritional needs.

A WORD FOR OPTIMISM

Both these stories bear witness to the preventive power of good nutrition, but they prove something that often goes without recognition. That's the support that comes from Shaklee people. The support comes in many forms, but it always adds up to an optimistic outlook.

An optimistic outlook is the ability to visualize yourself in better circumstances. It's an individual thing that only relates to you, but it works best when you have people supporting you. In Rosanna's life, it was a supportive husband; and in Phyllis' life, it was a soft-spoken friend who came into her life when she truly needed help.

18 Multiple Sclerosis

TODD'S STORY

"I was holding two jobs. We were saving money so we could buy a house and start our family." Todd was very energetic and didn't seem to tire, but every once in awhile his leg would seem to drag a little. He told himself that he needed more rest.

Rest didn't help and soon both his right arm and leg dragged. You would have thought that Todd was crippled or had had a stroke. Barb, his wife, took him to the hospital. From that day on their life would never be the same.

Many tests were done in the hospital. Doctors took blood, urine, x-rays, and magnetic imaging, which was a new technique in 1985. All this was followed by a spinal tap and a pronouncement: "Mike, you have multiple sclerosis. Judging from its progress, we believe you have had MS, as everyone calls it, for just over five years." The doctor, though gentle and understanding, was firm. He didn't mince words and explained that every test confirmed the diagnosis and there was no other possibility that he or anyone on the staff could offer. He told Todd that MS is progressive and would continue to develop and get worse as he got older. The medical approach is to try and get the MS to go into remission—become dormant—so you can continue with your life as well as possible. The doctor was very honest and clear, but held no hope for a cure; only for long periods of remission, at best.

WHAT IS MULTIPLE SCLEROSIS?

Multiple sclerosis means multiple scars, which in MS, appear on the nerves. The disease was discovered by a doctor who autopsied a woman who had unusual and diverse symptoms, which included all those that Mike had had, and more. She had kidney failure, bowel dysfunction, breathing difficulty, and other problems. The doctor found that her nerves had many scars; hence, the name, multiple sclerosis.

MS is an insidious disease that usually strikes between the ages of 20 and 40, although it is occasionally diagnosed around the age of 15. I say "insidious," because it develops slowly and without pain. Early symptoms are so minor that the victim usually isn't aware of anything wrong, much less that they have MS, until the disease has advanced. For example, the doctors concluded that Todd had MS for five years or more before its symptoms became obvious. His symptoms of fatigue and a dragging leg were typical.

MS is an inflammatory autoimmune-disease which attacks the central nervous system. That's a mouthful and I'll try and simplify it for you.

Autoimmune means that the body's immune system

treats some tissue as if it was a foreign invader and attacks it as if it was a threat. The tissue that is attacked — in MS it's nerve tissue — usually becomes inflamed. This is obvious in a disease like arthritis, but with MS, the inflammation goes unnoticed with the possible exception of minor neuropathy. Neuropathy is a loss of sensation in surface areas around the mouth or on the hands. To the victim, the feeling might seem like a slight tingling and is often ignored.

You might be wondering what causes the body's immune system to attack its own nerve tissue. There are no firm answers, but a pretty good hypothesis has developed from research. I'll take you through it so you'll see the tragedy of this terrible disease a little better.

Statistics show that MS prevails in temperate climates, such as the United States, at the rate of about 1 in 2,000 people compared to the Tropics, where 1 in 10,000 people get the disease. It favors women slightly over men, and seems to be slightly higher in some families. This slight edge to women and families doesn't mean it's inherited, because a virus seems to be involved. The climate distribution suggests more environmental factors that aren't clear at this time. However, it could be that the virus doesn't survive in warm climates.

Most experts suspect that a viral infection occurs many years before the symptoms and the virus either becomes dormant in nerve tissues or grows very slowly. This is based on the clear finding that people with MS have antibodies (immune factors) to viruses such as measles.

At some point in life the virus becomes active. Then to protect itself from the virus, the tissue — in MS it's the nerve tissue — becomes inflamed. Once the tissue is inflamed, the immune system dispatches cells which are supposed to attack the virus. For unknown reasons, these cells attack the body's own tissue, possibly attacking the virus at the same time. Perhaps it's a case of the good guys getting hit along with the bad guys.

In MS, the sheath around the nerve cells, the myelin sheath, is the specific tissue that's attacked. Think of the nerve as an electrical wire and the myelin sheath as the insulation around the electric wire. From experience, you know that serious problems, even disasters occur when insulation breaks down on the wires in your home or car. Well, it's the same in your body. You don't get fires and sparks in your body, but systems, such as kidneys, eyes, muscles, and other organs or tissue where nerves are important, break down. For example, the result of kidney failure can be death.

For a moment, I want to review what the hypothesis teaches about MS. First, the distribution of the disease means it's favored by cooler weather. The slight edge for women and families suggests there's a somewhat heightened susceptibility, but it's not as pronounced as an inflammatory disease like rheumatoid arthritis. This suggests a very slight predisposition, possibly to the virus.

Since MS fits some patterns of inflammatory diseases, we would expect stress, diet, fatigue, and nutrition to have a role in its development. Similar to other inflammatory diseases, we'd expect it to flare up and then enter periods of remission. MS can't be cured; all the victim can hope for is a long remission.

A flare-up leaves a scar on the nerve tissues that were attacked. Once enough scars have developed, you might lose most function in an organ or tissue. Historically, MS was called "creeping paralysis," because people with the disease would slowly lose the use of their legs or arms. MS victims often experience double vision, so the disease also affects the optic nerve and brain. Sometimes the sensory nerves are effected, so a part of your body might go numb. This is similar to having novocaine for dental work and then experiencing a "numb" mouth area.

With this as a background, let's trace Todd's experience and see how this disease emerges and how nutrition can help.

TODD NEEDS TWO CANES

Once released from the hospital, Todd needed two canes to walk. Here was a young man that had held two jobs; now he couldn't hold one and needed two canes just to get around. It was very depressing. He was put on a steroid regimen to help suppress the disease and get it into a dormant state. This meant constant constipation and regular discomfort.

Todd went to a cancer clinic that devoted some of its facilities to MS, with the objective of helping people cope with their illness. At the clinic he learned how to eat, so he would get enough fiber to stop the constipation. He was told to use food supplements to boost the nutrition his body needed. Most important, he met and commiserated with other MS victims at the clinic, and one person suggested he use Shaklee products.

After returning home, he used supplements from health-food stores and followed the dietary plan. His MS didn't get worse, but he still needed two canes to get around and he suffered with constant fatigue. He went to bed tired and woke up tired. After months of frustration, he decided to try Shaklee. He began with Vita-Lea, Instant Protein, Vita-E and a few other supplements. In a few days Todd noticed that he woke up feeling rested. He concluded that the Instant Protein did what people said: it gave him more energy, so he started taking it two times a day. Within nine months, he chucked the canes and decided to follow his plan for an education.

Once he had been diagnosed with MS, Todd decided he needed an education, so he applied to Purdue University for a grant. Though they didn't say the MS kept him out, they said: "Don't call us; we'll call you if we think there's a way you could get around." The call never came, but now he could walk into the administrative offices without canes and with the same vitality and energy everyone else had. He got the grant. Todd is now a college man who happens to have MS.

Todd is the first one to tell you he uses lots of supplements — Vita-Lea, Vita-E, B-Complex, and others. His twice daily standby is Instant Protein. For a man who needed two canes to just walk, he regularly drops the kids off on his way to school and pursues a twelve-hour day. His classes often mean lugging books up five flights of stairs. No problem. Evenings are spent sharing his nutrition knowledge at Shaklee meetings. This translates to carrying projectors, props, and displays. It's not unusual for him and Barb to return home after 11:00 p.m., but he's up again early the next morning to drop the kids on his way to school.

One of Todd's greatest rewards came from the silent joy he felt watching an embrace. It went like this. Todd speaks to MS support-groups about the value of good nutrition. Some people listen and some don't. For one couple, the disease had progressed to where they required wheelchairs, but they got married anyhow. After hearing Todd speak, they started the nutrition program that he followed. The special reward came one day when he saw this couple stand up in front of their wheelchairs to embrace. After the embrace, their conversation went like this: "Are you holding on?" "No, are you?" "No." They both cried. It was the first time they had kissed each other standing unassisted. No big deal for normal folks, but for them, it was a milestone that defies description.

Although Todd's experience with MS is typical, his was a mild, uncomplicated case compared to Janet's experience.

JANET'S STORY

"I couldn't see!" My mother took me to the eye doctor who hospitalized me immediately and called in a neurologist. The neurologist confirmed the eye-doctor's suspicion. Janet had MS. Married just two and a half years, 23-years-old, and she had a chronic illness that temporarily blinded her.

Once the MS went into remission, her vision returned. She went to a Catholic clinic in Tacoma, Washington where you learn to live with MS. What an experience. She saw MS in all its forms. There were people who couldn't walk or talk, some had kidney failure, and others couldn't even breathe. This taught Janet that any organ tissue and body function was fair game for MS. She made a vow: "It won't happen to me!"

Janet averaged two attacks each year; one around Christmas and the other at vacation time. MS attacks are precipitated by stress. It would take Janet about six months to recover from the attack, but each time the recovery restored a little less of the function that was affected. She was always left with a loss.

In spite of being told no children, she and her husband had a son six years after marriage. But the attacks continued and she developed a system of living. Janet learned how to ask others to help. Her husband did the grocery shopping, and her niece, whom they raised, did the housework.

A wheelchair was used whenever they went out. The wheelchair made it easier for other people. At home she used a cane. If a flare-up came, she learned to relax. She would get to bed and let her body heal itself.

Fatigue was her constant companion. This fatigue is called being "medically tired." Sleep doesn't change the feeling. Most people work hard, go to bed tired, and wake up refreshed. With MS you go to bed tired and wake up tired. It's like always dragging a dead weight—your body! Going out for an evening was a major ordeal. It meant resting the entire day. Then, the day after the outing was totally given over to rest.

A friend suggested she take Shaklee vitamins. She had read somewhere that vitamin E helps soften scar tissue, so she decided that would be the supplement to use. Her husband knew a man at work who sold Shaklee, so he picked some up for her. Janet then decided to read Adell Davis' book in which three-whole-pages were devoted to MS.

She started taking more supplements in addition to vitamin E: Vita-Lea, Vita-C, Instant Protein, and a few others. Nutrition is slow-motion medicine, and although the effects were accumulating, she was the last to notice. Friends who hadn't seen her in a long time said, "Janet, you look great. What are you doing?" Her husband wouldn't ask, "Are you too tired?" when someone suggested they stay for another round of bridge. Then one day she realized she was climbing stairs without a cane, like an adult and not a child.

Perhaps her greatest experience was a shopping trip. She went to a mall without a cane and not in a wheelchair, shopped for three hours, and left for home not feeling exhausted. She wasn't dragging a dead body anymore.

She started a Shaklee business to share her new health with others. In 5 years she had three, short flare-ups and hasn't had any for the past 15 years. On reflection, she realizes that the flare-ups occurred when she let her nutrition program fall. Her nutrition program includes: Instant Protein, Vita-Lea, B-Complex, Vita-C, Vita-E, Beta Carotene, Alfalfa, and Calcium. Janet also uses one or two Herb-Lax daily to keep her regularity.

She describes herself as an MS sufferer in recovery. Janet realizes the disease is there waiting to flare up if she lets her guard down.

CAROL'S STORY

I met Carol while speaking in Canada. She remarked that she has MS, but was saved by nutrition. I asked her to tell me her story. It is very much like Janet's and Todd's story, with a major exception. Carol's kidneys stopped working.

She said, "I could tolerate the wheelchair and the canes, but a month on dialysis twice a week and I considered letting God have me." Then some friends suggested she start a nutrition program. At first her doctor balked at the idea, but then relented and said, "You can't get worse."

Carol took Vita-Lea, Instant Protein, Vita-E, and Vita-C. Within a couple of weeks, about 10 percent of her kidney function reappeared. This wasn't expected. She persisted and after another month she was off dialysis. Within six months she didn't require a wheelchair. She still uses a cane, and for long sessions out she'll go in a wheelchair, so she can get around faster. It's just more practical.

Carol's story of fatigue is right out of the book, with one exception. She said it like this. "It's not just physical fatigue, it's also mental. You reach a point where you don't care about living. The only reason you go on is because your body won't die."

IS THIS IN THEIR HEADS?

Did Todd, Janet, and Carol experience mind over disease? No, but the support of an optimistic group around them helped. MS is a terrible disease. When a nerve is attacked it can either block a motor function like walking, a kidney function, a sensory function like vision or feeling, or a combination of these functions. That's real. It can be measured.

Medical fatigue is real, not imagined. It results from the incredible stress on the body, that an attack on the nervous system precipitates. Just because you sleep, the attack doesn't stop. Three processes are constantly taking place. The body is being attacked; it's trying to defend itself; and it's trying to repair its systems. When a nerve fails in one part of the body, it effects the entire system.

Chronic fatigue, a constant symptom of MS, is a clue

that there's a common denominator to it all. The body is fighting under constant stress to repair a vital system. This fight calls for big-league nourishment with all the nutrients. No one knows what the requirements are for a person with MS. Suffice to say, just getting the RDA of nutrients can't possibly be enough. Besides, each person is as different as they look and as the systems that MS attacks.

WHAT CAN WE LEARN FROM THIS?

MS is one of the most insidious diseases of our time. Science tells us that it has similarities to other autoimmune diseases, and that somewhere a virus seems to remain dormant until it flares up and causes the body to attack its own nervous tissues.

Like other inflammatory diseases, it seems to flare up when the victim is under stress. Stress brings some changes that include a drop in some nutrients, such as vitamin C and some of the B vitamins. But it also brings changes in the immune system. We know this from experience that your mother probably expressed: "You caught a cold because you were rundown."

We also know from research, that in addition to the usual vitamins and minerals, vitamin E is essential to nerve cells. It's an important part of those cells and the myelin sheath, and is essential to their function. This pattern is confirmed by the rare instances where we can study a vitamin-E deficiency. I believe that MS creates an extraordinary need for vitamin E. EPA also falls into the same category.

Protein serves two functions: tissue repair and energy. Instant Protein is uniquely suited for this purpose. So not surprising, when people with MS start the use of protein, they seem to recover more quickly and the fatigue slowly disappears.

Diet can probably help MS. The diet should be low in animal fat, and rich in fish, vegetables and fruit. A diet such as the one I wrote in *The Arthritis Relief Diet* would be prudent. A good supplement program is essential.

19 PMS Premenstrual Syndrome

NAN'S STORY

"Hell came once a month," she said. Nan is a young woman under 30, with a great job, who lived with a common disorder that has no known cause and certainly no accepted cure. The disorder is called premenstrual syndrome (PMS).

"I call it 'hell' because I felt terrible, and I made sure everyone else around me felt terrible, as well." Nan explained exactly how she felt every month when she had PMS.

She would experience a dull ache in her abdomen about three days before her period. As the day approached, she would feel crampy, bloated, and sick. Although she often didn't realize it, she would be aggressively irritable and abrupt with family, friends, and co-workers. Invariably, Nan would miss at least one day of work each month. If she didn't miss work, it was because the "sick day" was on a Saturday, Sunday, or holiday.

"I would go to the doctor about it several times each

year," she laughed. Nan tried all sorts of things recommended for PMS ranging from simple aspirin, stronger analgesics, and some steroid therapy, to PMS tea she bought in a health-food store, special herbs, and so on. Some relief would come, but things would get out of synchrony. Nan explains it well: "I'd feel terrible, call the doctor, and get to see her the next day. By then I'd feel miserable, so the doctor would try things to relieve the symptoms, but they never eliminated the disorder. They would usually work to some degree, but only to ease the symptoms."

Sometimes her PMS would skip a month or two, or it wouldn't be as bad, so Nan would escape the ordeal temporarily. But then it would return. After awhile you get desperate, and so do the people you live and work with. "Believe me, it was a dreaded part of the month and I just wished it would go away. After awhile I would warn my family and friends that it was that time of the month, so it was best to just avoid me. They didn't have to be told twice."

"Diuretics seemed to help if I started taking them about a week before my period." The diuretic her doctor prescribed kept her fluid retention down, so the bloating was milder and somewhat of a relief. But it didn't seem to stop the anxiety, irritability, and malaise that came.

JEAN'S STORY

Jean is a mother of two boys, now aged 23 and 21. That makes them men, but to her they'll always be boys. Jean had PMS since she can remember. When she was 17 her PMS was so bad that she tore a bed sheet lengthwise down the middle, while laying in bed trying to get past the cramps. You can imagine the intensity of the pain she must have experienced, as it's not easy to tear a bed sheet unless it's very old.

"My doctor thought the PMS would clear after my first child was born. It did until about six months after I stopped nursing," she said and continued. "It wasn't as bad after that, but I would still get it and everyone around me got it as well."

After her second son was born, Jean figured her PMS would finally go. Once again, she started getting PMS a few months after she stopped nursing. So much for her doctor's theory that childbirth was some kind of great equalizer. Jean had become convinced that she'd be dogged by PMS until menopause. And if her luck with childbirth was any indicator, she was wary of that as well. Besides, she had heard that after menopause, doctors prescribed steroids to avoid getting osteoporosis later in life. After all she had been through, she decided osteoporosis would be better than PMS.

NAN AND JEAN TRY REMEDIES

Both these women, though far apart in years, had tried the same things for their problem. They had never met each other; they had just read the same articles in newspapers and magazines, and the same books on the subject. Both women had tried taking B6, magnesium, and even black cohosh, an herb that looks, smells, and tastes gross. They would often believe they were onto something that worked, but success would vanish like the morning mist.

Like many other women, they independently tried a special diet for the problem. They felt better. It was a good diet and they lost a little weight, even if they didn't need to lose any. Many times they heaved a sigh of relief, thinking their life-long problem was solved. Not so. The curse of the devil always returned.

Jean even found an exercise group for women who had menstrual problems. She felt better about herself for exercising and was convinced it helped. Both women exercise regularly today. However, at that time, they usually had to skip a few days of exercise during that time of the month.

NUTRITION

Independently, each woman came to use Shaklee products. Jean went to a nutrition seminar with a friend and Nan heard about it from a girl at work. They both went on a full nutrition program that included protein, Vita-Lea, B-Complex, vitamin E, calcium-magnesium, Herb-Lax, and other supplements.

After several months of freedom from PMS, they were both stuck in a dilemma. Was it one product or several products that were making the difference? They experimented by eliminating various products, with the exception of Vita-Lea.

Several products seemed to have a definite influence on them, but two seemed to be outstanding: B-Complex and vitamin E, which they took in addition to Vita-Lea. They know that if they eliminate either one for a month, the PMS returns. Even though they take the products, they both seem to get some symptoms every month.

Since Nan and Jean started using Shaklee products, some new products have appeared: beta carotene and EPA. Now they use both of these products regularly. However, both women insist that vitamin E and B-Complex are their standbys.

Over the years these women have learned that Herb-Lax and Fiber Blend help relieve the bloating, and they've tried alfalfa with success. However, they both keep referring back to their old standbys.

WHAT GOES ON HERE?

PMS is one of the most elusive of all human ailments. It comes and goes each month or so. You'd think that medicine would be able to conquer it. But unfortunately, it's not so easy.

Much of PMS is subjective, so you have to find women who have the problem, get them to follow a regimen or take a drug regularly for several months, at least, and then crossover to placebo pills or regimen. It's not very easy, considering they also have to hold jobs, go to school, or raise kids during that time. After all, it's not an illness that confines them to a hospital. In spite of the above difficulties, research has produced some consistent results.

While attending an American College of Nutrition meeting in 1988, I became interested in PMS. A paper was presented, in which the researchers showed that vitamin E had a positive influence on PMS. I've been following this research ever since and have looked into past research.

Four nutrients seem to consistently produce positive results: the B-Complex of vitamins, vitamin E, gamma linolenic acid (GLA), and calcium. GLA is usually obtained from evening primrose oil or black-currant seed oil, although there are other sources. A recent study showed that calcium produced positive results at about 1,300-milligrams daily.

Results are never clear. Some trials produce positive results and all produce mixed results. But the trend for the above four nutrients have a consistently positive direction.

Regular exercise and good diet also helps. This suggests that other factors go awry that exaggerate the PMS. Surely these other factors include swings in blood sugar, fluid retention, and constipation. Lack of regularity, usually constipation, seems to exaggerate any health problem.

My conclusions are that diet, supplements, and exercise are critical to keeping PMS symptoms to a minimum. Diet should emphasize "high" fiber, complex carbohydrates, moderate stimulants, and no high-sugar snacks.

Supplements should be based around Vita-Lea, B-Complex, vitamin E, and calcium-magnesium. Gamma linolenic acid (GLA) should also be a serious consideration. Fiber and Herb-Lax for occasional irregularity seem correct, as well.

You will hear that other supplements help or are essential. I'm sure they do help, and for some people are essential. For example, virtually everyone I know derives some benefit from protein and vitamin C. However, I'm not sure that any additional supplements will specifically help relieve PMS.

CHAPTER

20 Stuttering

SUE'S STORY

"Stuttering makes you tired. Saying anything becomes hard work," Sue said. Then I commented that it's also tiring for the person who does the listening. As I talked to this pretty, friendly lady who enjoyed conversation, I couldn't believe she had been a severe stutterer. She talks about so many things. She continued, "From the time I was a little girl until I was a teenager, I couldn't put three words together. It took me five minutes to say something another person could say in 30 seconds." No matter how you see it, that's serious stuttering.

Sue did what any other young girl should do that can't stop stuttering, she didn't speak much. In her words, "I learned how to get along in school without ever raising my hand in class. I'd have to get a point across with one word. I could go to a birthday party or play with other children and never speak a word. If you think about it, it's no different than a child who has a bad leg or hand; they learn how to get around in spite of their handicap. Well,

I learned to get along without speaking more than one or two words at a time."

When I thought about what Sue said, I had to agree. I realized that when I speak with people who stutter, I become impatient and try to complete their sentences for them. It makes me tired to listen to them. When I think about stuttering, I realize how tough it must be for the person who stutters. How tired they must get.

For me, stuttering would be like living out a bad dream; one where you know what you want to say, but the words won't come out. To overcome her handicap, Sue mastered other skills in school. She developed excellent dexterity, learned to write well, and became very expressive with her hand and body language. Sue is good at doing things. I guess a child who stutters has to be a doer, and not an explainer. I asked Sue if her parents had sought medical help to cure the stuttering.

"Medical help? I saw every speech therapist within a thousand miles. If a school had a speech center, I went there. Anyone who had the slightest glimmer of knowledge about speech got a call from my parents. I spent 13 years in speech therapy with no summer vacation." Sue can laugh about it now, but you can imagine how difficult it must have been for her.

When you look at Sue it's easy to see that being especially pretty made the situation worse. Somehow, people expect a person with an impediment to look different than everyone else. They aren't expected to be the prettiest girl in the class.

"I was even sent to a medical hypnotist." A medical hypnotist uses hypnosis to correct something that's in your head. They help some people who stutter; they do a lot for children who don't have bladder control; they help people stop smoking; and they help people eliminate tics and twitches. "But," Sue said, "he didn't help me one bit. In fact, he told me I even stuttered under hypnosis. I think his efforts, to no avail, helped my parents accept my stuttering as part of me. I'm Sue and I stutter." When I reflected on what she said, I could understand the dilemma her parents faced. She was doing nicely with an impediment, but they wanted to help her. We often don't realize that people born with an impediment learn to live with it, because they don't know any other way of living.

If a child is born with a deformed or missing limb, you accept it. Somehow we accept the fact that people can't grow new arms or legs, so they go on with life from there. But if all the doctors examine your stuttering child and say she's normal, what are you supposed to do? Since her speech apparatus—voice box, tongue, and so on—is normal, you conclude there's something awry in her head, so you go to a neurologist.

Then, if the neurologist does the brain scans and nerve-system tests and says she's normal, you're left with but one conclusion: it's psychosomatic. Consequently, you try the therapists, hypnotists, and positive thinkers. When none of that works, you slowly stop trying, because by that time your little girl is now your big girl, and she's getting along just fine.

Sue finished high school, went on to college, and met a handsome young man. Biology took over for Ray and Sue, and they soon got married. Both of them had excellent careers and eventually started a family. Sue had adapted very well to her speech impediment and had learned to make her wishes known without saying much verbally. She would use body language with a word or two, and got along just fine.

Sue started using Shaklee products because a friend was selling them. She started with the usual product grouping of protein, Vita-Lea, vitamin C, calcium, and an Herb-Lax or two. She noticed that she had more energy. "One thing stuttering does is make you tired. Once I started on Shaklee, I noticed I wasn't tired any longer. I didn't need naps. This prompted me to start experimenting with other products."

"I used vitamins E and C, tried the skin-care products, and even used the household products," she said. "One day, I took some B-complex. If I remember correctly, I took one or two with each meal every day. After about a week, my speech seemed smoother." She talked about this experience as if it was yesterday, when it was actually over 15 years ago.

"Ray commented that my speech seemed smoother. I also noticed that it wasn't the same hard work to put a long sentence together. Since I had added only B-complex to my daily regimen, I decided to increase the amount. I took three B-complex at each meal and three more at bed-time. A day of this plan and my stuttering just about stopped immediately." Sue talks about it with detachment, but is quick to point out, "At the time it seemed too good to be true. It was like an enormous weight lifted off my shoulders. I felt like dancing in the streets."

She experimented with B-complex after that. If she stopped B-complex, the stuttering returned. By trial and error, Sue found that four B-complex at each meal and four more before going to bed is an optimum amount. "I could probably get by with three, but four makes me feel safe, so why not?"

IS THIS IN HER HEAD?

I guess you'd have to say "yes," because the speech centers are definitely part of your brain. If you have a normal voice box, tongue, and so on, it has to be in your brain. But that's evading the point. What we really want to know is if her use of B-Complex to stop the stuttering is some sort of psychological issue, mind over matter, or wishful thinking? I think Sue proved it's not by testing herself. And if you said it was only mental, how would you explain everything else?

Sue went through 13 years of formal speech therapy, besides seeing psychologists, psychiatrists, neurologists, and a medical hypnotist. That's the equivalent of going from kindergarten through high school. If wishful thinking could have solved Sue's problem, it would have been solved.

A few years ago, some research was published on people who stuttered. The paper pointed out that parts of the brain of stutterers don't have good blood circulation. I guess that says it's a developmental deficiency. By itself, that observation doesn't prove anything about Sue, but if you add to that her experience, you can speculate on what went on with her.

Four B-complex tablets provide eighteen times the RDA for the B vitamins, except for folic acid and biotin, for which the four tablets provide four times the RDA. This amount of B-Complex totals over 636 milligrams of physiologically-active materials and could shift normal B-vitamin levels far enough from their normal level positions to change metabolic rates or increase circulation to the extremities. By taking four B-Complex four-times daily, Sue maintains these high RDA levels consistently with the exception of a few hours at night when she's sleeping. But as she pointed out, she has sort of settled on a slight excess, so her use probably compensates for this period of time as well.

Most of us don't think of our head as an extremity, but from a circulatory or metabolic point of view, our head is an extremity. Our head and hands are usually the only extremities exposed to the environment.

Most body heat is lost or actively dissipated through the head and hands. You know from experience, that when it's cold outside, a hat often keeps you warmer than an extra sweater. Similarly for nice warm mittens. Many people observe this similar effect from B-Complex without knowing it. They notice an improvement in fingernail growth. Folks often tell me their nails and even hair are stronger. It may surprise you, but fingernails are a kind of specialized hair. Protein will cause the same effect, called thermogenesis, as B-Complex. Old-time scientists refer to it as "specific dynamic action."

So if some experts are correct about brain circulation in some people who stutter, and that it's related to, if not causing the stuttering, then Sue happened onto a solution that works for her. Will it work for other people? Who knows? I think it's worth a try. Perhaps someday a researcher will be able to get enough volunteers and financial support to rigorously study the phenomenon under clinical conditions.

One thing is certain, nothing else ever worked for Sue. And what makes her correction of the stuttering even more relevant, is that she wasn't searching for a solution. It wasn't even on her mind. She had learned to live with stuttering as if it was normal. By any measure, Sue was very successful in life and didn't need to solve what, to her, had ceased being a problem. This makes her story that much more important.

21 When No One Knows

Did you ever have a car that didn't run right and mechanics couldn't find the source of the trouble? First, it was a new fuel pump; then an electronic gadget; at another time it was air getting into the fuel line; next, a short in the spark-plug wire, and so on. Finally, in desperation, you conclude your car's a lemon. You make do and quit taking it to the mechanic. You decide to keep driving it until it stops dead, or until you become so frustrated you buy a new car.

Many times the same thing happens to people. But they can't trade in their body. They've got to get along with the only one they will ever have.

LORENE'S STORY

Lorene is now 59, as I try to recapture her conversion to nutrition. Her story starts when she was about 45-years-old. She has five children and couldn't remember ever being really sick, other than having an occasional cold or flu. Being the mother of a large family just didn't leave time to be sick. Outside of the usual childhood ailments that most kids get, her children, two boys and three girls, were generally healthy, as well.

Lorene's problems started one spring when she got headaches off and on every few days. At first she thought it was simply changes in the weather. Then she did what most people do, she took aspirin and the headaches seemed to clear up. Or, as she put it, "Maybe I'd just forget them because I was always so busy. However, the headaches persisted and I didn't like taking aspirin all the time, so I went to our family doctor."

The doctor couldn't find anything wrong with Lorene. He explained that the headaches weren't migraines or cluster headaches, so he said to get more rest and continue using aspirin, when necessary. He didn't prescribe anything stronger because her headaches weren't that bad. Consequently, she simply learned to live with the headaches and use aspirin.

After awhile Lorene started to feel nauseated in the mornings and very tired when she got up. She knew she wasn't pregnant, so she went back to the doctor. He told her to use antacids. Unfortunately, they were no cure. The queasy stomach persisted and Lorene continued to feel tired. This lasting stomach problem led the doctor to suspect an ulcer, so he put her through an upper GI series. It was a terrible ordeal, but it showed that she didn't have an ulcer. The tests didn't find anything indicative.

A negative diagnosis didn't make her feel better. Indeed, she felt more frustrated because she didn't feel right, but was told she was fine. Canker sores began appearing in her mouth. They would come and go, but they hurt. She used things to relieve the pain and conceal the sores, but they still came; probably, she thought, because she was run down and tired. She started going to bed earlier so she could get more sleep, and had the children do more of the work around the house. "Somehow, sleeping longer just made me feel more tired," she said.

Depression reared its ugly head. Between headaches, a queasy stomach, and the coming and going of canker sores, her life seemed to be going downhill. Face it, with her children being more independent, she seemed to feel less and less needed. "One day I started crying for no apparent reason," she said. "I was sitting at the table over coffee one minute and crying in my coffee the next." This lead to another visit to the doctor, who decided to run some thyroid tests. Nothing. Then, she had a glucose-tolerance test, which turned out normal. Somehow, between the testing and the doctors, she started thinking she was really sick. The next thing she noticed was red blotches, like a rash, but without pimples, on her stomach and chest. They didn't hurt, but they looked like they should hurt. Lorene felt miserable.

"All this time I'd get a headache during the day that would last for an hour or so. I'd lay down and it would leave, but then I'd feel worn out. If a cold or flu went around, I'd get it along with everyone else. I wouldn't be any worse than my friends, but it would linger at a low level. Or rather than linger, it would come back." Lorene would start feeling better and then be knocked down again. It was as if her body would recover just so far and stop.

I asked her if her weight went up or down. She said, "no," but she recognized that she got puffy, felt tired, and actually gained a pound or two around the time of her period each month. I asked her if she had regular bowel movements. She observed that she never felt constipated, and had a movement every few days. An accepted normal level is one bowel movement in 24- to 36-hours.

Lorene experienced low-back pain one month when she got her period. The pain wasn't severe, like a slipped disc or even a sprain, which she had had, but it never seemed to leave. Most mothers have had a back sprain at one time or another and know what they're like. This pain was just a dull ache that wasn't there when she woke up, but appeared about mid-morning after she had been on her feet for awhile. "Sometimes I would take a coffee break with a neighbor and get up from the table with a low-back pain. Then this nagging ache would persist until I went to bed."

This back ache called for another trip to the doctor. He was reluctant to x-ray because he didn't think it was a disc problem. He said it was a sprain. "You're getting older," he said, "and have to slow down." The doctor gave her a prescription for muscle relaxants, and told her to take one when the pain came. "I took the medication a few times and it would work, but I was reluctant to use it daily. I found myself just taking them at night to sleep," she said.

Lorene made an appointment with her gynecologist, thinking she had "female problems." The doctor couldn't find anything wrong, but in her judgment, Lorene's problems could be early menopause. After running a series of blood tests, that proved Lorene was quite normal, the doctor concluded the problems would resolve themselves as she went through menopause. Even though it was comforting to think she would grow out of the problems, Lorene felt the best years of her life slipping by in a state of "not feeling good." Lorene felt depressed either because of the illness, or because no one could find an illness. Even though her children were fine and her husband had a good job, her outlook was not optimistic. She found herself looking at things in a negative way. When she looked in the mirror, the face looking back didn't sparkle. Her complexion had become gray, she had dark bags under her dull eyes, and her hair had no luster. She would become most upset when people asked her what was wrong. They could tell by looking at her that something wasn't right. She couldn't give a definite answer, so every friend recommended a doctor "who was marvelous." Lorene tried going to some of these doctors and was poked, probed, tested, and tested again. Usually the diagnosis was vague, like "you're entering your change of life," or "have you ever seen a psychiatrist?"

A friend asked Lorene to try some Shaklee products and attend a seminar put on by Barbara Lagoni. The seminar motivated her to try a basic routine of Vita Lea, Instant Protein, and Herb-Lax. Lorene felt better at the end of the first week. She started having a bowel movement every day. "I seemed to loose my puffiness." In less than ten days she noticed a difference in the mirror. Her eyes were clear and the bags were gone. Her complexion took on a rosy glow; it didn't look gray anymore.

After the second week her headaches stopped. "I didn't realize it until one day I just noticed how good I felt." She had the same energy she had years ago and didn't feel tired at 9:30 in the evening. Lorene's outlook improved. She became more optimistic and less cynical. One day she ran into a friend in the supermarket. "Lorene, you look great! What have you been doing to yourself?"

Lorene sticks with the Shaklee plan that includes Vita

Lea, Instant Protein, B-complex, Vita-C, Calcium-Magnesium, and one or two Herb-Lax. Sometimes she uses lots of other products, but sticks to this basic plan— her "standby." She openly says that if she deviates from this plan, she can feel depression coming on. In fact, she claims her depression is stopped by taking B-Complex.

The low-back pain seemed to disappear when she was about six- or seven-months into her supplement program. The pain didn't just stop all at once, it seemed to slowly disappear. She still has a bottle of muscle relaxers just in case anyone needs them.

IS IT IN HER HEAD?

Of course not. Lots of people go for a long time not feeling well. They can make repeated visits to their doctor and still not come up with anything specific. When doctors can't find anything wrong, it's usually because the tests they've ordered have eliminated serious problems and the remaining possibilities are nebulous, at best. It's like nailing Jello to a tree. Sometimes the problem is diet related, brought on by too much stress, working too hard, or something else. It's hard for anyone to track these type of ailments to their source.

Often these problems feed on each other. Your complexion looks poor, so you worry. Worry creates all kinds of non-specific problems, which get you depressed. I call this frustrating stage of the dilemma the "downward spiral," because one thing finds the other and it gets progressively worse. Ultimately, these things lead to a psychologist's couch.

Not surprisingly, Lorene's nutrition program had a

powerful influence on her health. Regularity and a good complexion go together like milk and honey. Good metabolism and an optimistic outlook can't be separated. Indeed, I truly believe optimism or pessimism reflects what's going on inside our body.

In support of my hypothesis, think of this: Any nutritional shortfall shows up first in the brain. A review of the classical cases of scurvy, or the famous B-vitamin deficiencies, proves that these deficiencies show up first in the mind. Indeed, depression or dullness always precede other symptoms. We have a tendency to discount mental outlook, however, because it's so vague. Who hasn't had a headache, felt depressed, been cynical, anxious, and so on? We simply don't think of these eventualities as important, unless they're so bad that they're obvious. Then we turn to medication first; not food.

Low-back pain is the first sign of osteoporosis. Classic double-blind studies first done by Doctor Anthony Albanese, showed that as bone density is restored, low-back pain often disappears. This is because the backbone is one of the first bones to lose its density when calcium is short. However, it takes about six- or more-months for this to happen. Most people look for an immediate solution to their pain. They never think about the years it took for their problem to develop, and that it might take at least a few months for it to disappear. Lorene's experience fits this pattern like a hand and glove.

In addition, as we get older and live under even increasing stress, our nutrient requirements increase. When we get minor ailments like Lorene described, we need more of most nutrients and don't get them.

Now add to that a recent dietary analysis of American's habits that appeared in the December 1990, *American*

Journal of Public Health. In brief, it shows that about 9 percent of us regularly eat a balanced diet. Then, in the same month, the *American Journal of Epidemiology* pointed out that only 23.1 percent of adults use supplements consistently. Worse, 51.1 percent of adults use supplements intermittently. This means that our diets aren't balanced, and we aren't consistent enough with supplements to make up the shortfalls. Actually, the papers show that most people take the wrong supplements anyhow.

How often have you heard someone say, "I'm tired. I think I'll have another cup of coffee," in contrast to, "I'm tired. I need better nutrition, exercise and more sound sleep."?

Lorene described, quite clearly, the outcome of a good nutrition program: energy, a good complexion, an optimistic outlook, and sound sleep. Then add to that list the absence of vague problems, like too many canker sores, colds that seem to come back, or thinking your skin is gray. It all fits a pattern that usually clears when a person takes control of their nutrition.

Afterword

In my need for brevity, I had to restrict the number of stories I selected for this book. I only wanted to make a point, and more stories would have been redundant. First, I wanted to capture the value that super nutrition plays in seemingly unrelated health-problems, and then I wanted people to see the Shaklee spirit at work.

Research has proven, more than once, that people succeed better at anything they attempt when they're in a supportive environment. Indeed, a study on terminal cancer patients, conducted by Stanford Medical School, proved the value of a positive outlook. In this famous study, one group of terminal cancer patients was coached in developing an optimistic outlook by people trained in positive thinking. The other group of terminal patients was similar in every aspect, except it was given books to read on a positive approach without any coaching. In short, they were simply left on their own. The group who got the support of people, lived, on average, eighteen months longer than the control group.

None of us would even want to be in either group.

However, it's from these exaggerated research situations that truths come to the surface. An optimistic outlook, human support, fellowship, knowing someone cares, and most important, having someone say "you can do it," help us to thrive when we might have just survived. In the Stanford study, the support provided a longer life.

Most of us never get a round of applause after we graduate from high school, and we don't always get one then. Most of us never have the advantage of a supportive group, yet it's nice to have people around who are supportive of the things we try to accomplish. Sure, our family is supportive, but too often we take their support for granted, or it's too quiet for us to hear. Family support isn't usually appreciated until we're older and can realize how deep love goes.

Shaklee people learn, by experience, not to hear the abundance of negatives in life. This positive outlook slowly invades the very being of their personality and takes over their spirit. Because of this outlook, Shaklee meetings are positive and optimistic. As a group, these individuals look for the good qualities in people and search for the silver lining in each gray cloud. Optimism is their watchword.

Because of this all pervasive, positive outlook, the people, whose stories I told in this book, were nurtured in an optimistic environment. While these people were going through their period of travail, they were being coached to find any positive signs, no matter how subtle they might be. As a result, I suspect they persisted with their maximum nutrition effort, while others, left on their own, would have quit. Perseverance is the foundation of all success.

An axiom teaches that success comes from what you do

when no one is looking. Think of the endless hours of practice that make the successful concert pianist; the adherence to a standard of excellence that drives the artist to capture the right essence in his or her paintings; the number of unpublished books that makes the successful writer; and a careful, constant honing of ethics that lets the politician grow into a statesman. Similarly with successful Shaklee people. Their continual, careful cultivation of a positive attitude must go on 24-hours daily for them to succeed.

However, the optimism comes together in one simple concept: "You help yourself by helping others," which is an expression of the Shaklee philosophy. This attitude is the basis of many success stories, and especially the ones in this book. If a distributor somewhere didn't persist in offering unwavering support, none of the people in this book would have succeeded. The foundation of sharing, the basis of the Golden Rule, is absolutely essential for success.

LAUGH AT YOURSELF

I noticed that Shaklee folks, like all of us, make mistakes. After all, to err is human. But Shaklee folks seem to be able to laugh at themselves when they make a mistake or blunder. This, I've decided, is a very important quality.

Most of us take life seriously. After all, it's tough to stay where you are, let alone get ahead. However, most of us also take ourselves seriously and that's not necessarily good. You can identify this trait first in the teacher, who's the authority in the room and is always "right."

When you're the expert on everything all day, it's tough to realize you're not the dominant power once the bell rings.

We see this same trait in the star athlete whose talent takes them to the top. Next thing you know, they are asked to appear everywhere. No one ever tells them, "You're just another guy with an extraordinary talent that can fade, so what often happens is that they "crash" mentally when a new star comes along. While they were riding high, they took themselves too seriously.

This same trait is sometimes more obvious in the business executive who, while smart, clever, and wise, often forgets that much of his success has come from being in the right place at the right time. In other words, luck. He also forgets that all the sycophants that surround him are being paid partially to make him look good and partially to massage his ego. After awhile, he begins to be a universal authority on everything and believes his own rhetoric. Then, when his position is gone, he wonders where his friends are. He took himself too seriously.

I could go on and on with examples. We're all important and yet we're all unimportant. Consequently, when we make a blunder, the world doesn't care and neither should we. It's important to realize that no one knows everything or is even correct half of the time. You've only got to be correct once to succeed. So, when you make a mistake, laugh at it, and the world will laugh with you.

HUMOR

Another aspect of Shaklee life is humor. These people learn to see humor in everyday things. This lightens life and lets them go through life with a smile. After all, laughter is a form of medicine, because when you're laughing, your mind isn't thinking of heavy things. It, too, is laughing.

VISUALIZATION

A second element of optimism—perhaps the very essence of optimism for people—is self visualization. You must be able to visualize yourself as healthy in order to be healthy. This doesn't mean that doctors, drugs, surgery, or nutrition aren't necessary. It means that personal outlook and optimism is part of your success. I've heard doctors talk about how a person's "will to live" kept them alive; or how a "lack of will" let them die. Outlook made the difference. This is just another way of saying: "He saw himself or herself as living through their travail and growing healthy. More importantly, they never wavered from that vision."

To succeed at anything requires seeing yourself as successful. Visualization pervades every aspect of life and health.

DIET: AN UNSUNG PARTNER

These nutritional success stories give credit to the Shaklee supplements. But in each case I studied, I could see how the people involved also improved their diet, which is as much a part of the Shaklee program as an optimistic outlook. Total health becomes infectious.

At first I noticed how many people would eliminate red meat, white flour, or soft drinks from their diet. They started reading books on nutrition. Their diets became good, then very good, and they passed the concepts on to their family, friends, and almost anyone who would listen to them expound. Without knowing it, they became consumed by holistic health.

Supplements depend on a good diet for support; they go hand and hand. Without a good diet, the best supplements will not produce their best results. As Doctor Shaklee explained, food supplements are meant to supplement food—good, natural food. This brings one last thought to the fore.

HARMONY WITH NATURE

Experts say that about 80 percent of most human illnesses will clear up by themselves. Unsaid in this statement is that this natural healing depends on complete nutrition, an optimistic outlook, and the right lifestyle. In a few words: living in harmony with nature.

Living in harmony with nature means you've got to practice the concepts of good health 24 hours a day. These are things you do when no one is looking. Success in health, like success in anything, is a full-time commitment.

Complete nutrition means a good diet and the correct supplements. It includes pure water, clean air, a variety of natural foods, and correct moderation in all of them.

An optimistic outlook teaches that we must use the past to make a better future. Therefore, we should use blunders as lessons in what not to do. Emphasis must always be placed on being better and setting realistic goals.

Spiritual nutrition goes beyond human fellowship. Spiritual nourishment requires intellectual questioning of where we came from and where we're going. It can't be obtained without exercising our mind to seek answers to these fundamental questions.

Lifestyle is almost common sense. A good lifestyle has the obvious elements of exercise, and moderation in pleasure. But it also means that we need to be able to laugh at ourselves, take criticism from a well-intended friend, and share our ideas with other.

It appears to me that we humans also require love. It's as if we have to share love to be complete. All love begins with respect. We must respect life, ourselves, and see beyond the flaws. Once we can look past the flaws, we can find unquestioned love. Once we give love without conditions, we can receive the love, trust, and respect of others. With love, our lives will be complete and we'll truly live in harmony with nature.

ABOUT THE AUTHOR

James Scala was educated at Columbia (B.A.), Cornell (Ph.D.), and Harvard (Post-doctoral studies) Universities.

He has spent his career in research, research management, and teaching. His accomplishments include over fifty published papers on research in nutrition, biochemistry, and biology. His teaching includes courses for undergraduate, graduate, medical, and dental school students.

As a research manager, Dr. Scala held positions at Procter and Gamble, Owens-Illinois, Unilever, General Foods, and was the Senior Vice-President of Scientific Affairs for the Shaklee Corporation. He now devotes his energies to writing and speaking for the general public.

Dr. Scala lives with his wife Nancy in Lafayette, California. For recreation, they sail the ketch La Scala from its home port on San Francisco Bay.

OTHER BOOKS BY DR. SCALA

Making the Vitamin Connection, Harper and Row, 1985.

The Arthritis Relief Diet, NAL, 1988.

The High Blood Pressure Relief Diet, NAL, 1989.

Eating Right For A Bad Gut, NAL, 1990.

Look 10 Years Younger, Feel 10 Years Better, Piatkus, 1991. Co-authored with Barbara Jacques.

Prescription For Longevity, E.P. Dutton, March 1992.

Technical Books:

Nutritional Determinants in Athletic Performance, edited with Drs. Haskel and Whittam.

New Protective Effects of Some Unique Nutrients, edited with Dr. Gene Spiller.

Better Health Series Books:

Food Supplements for High Blood Pressure

Healthy Skin, Nails, Hair, and Eyes

How to Add Years to Your Life and Life to Your Years

Lower Your Cholesterol in 30 days

Nourishing Healthy Children

Supplementation in Arthritis